Diagnosis in color

Physical Signs in General Medicine

second edition

Michael Zatouroff
FRCP Lond.

Physician
The London Clinic
London W1

Hon Senior Lecturer
Academic Department of Medicine
Royal Free Hospital
London

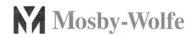 Mosby-Wolfe

London • Baltimore • Barcelona • Bogotá • Boston
Buenos Aires • Carlsbad, CA • Chicago • Madrid
Mexico City • Milan • Naples, FL • New York
Philadelphia • St. Louis • Seoul • Singapore
Sydney • Taipei • Tokyo • Toronto • Wiesbaden

Publisher:	**Richard Furn**
Development Editor:	**Jennifer Prast**
Project Manager:	**Paul Phillips**
Production:	**Jane Tozer**
Index:	**Anita Reid**
Design:	**Lara Last**
Cover Design:	**Greg Smith**

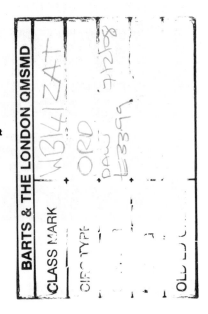

Copyright © 1996 Times Mirror International Publishers Limited

Published in 1996 by Mosby, an imprint of Times Mirror International Publishers Limited

Printed by Grafos, S.A. ARTE SOBRE PAPEL

ISBN   Hardback: 0 7234 2326 1

Softback: 0 7234 2587 6

For full details of all Times Mirror International Publishers Limited titles, please write to Times Mirror International Publishers Limited, Lynton House, 7–12 Tavistock Square, London WC1H 9LB, England.

A CIP catalogue record for this book is available from the British Library.

Diagnosis i

Physical Signs in General Medicine

second edition

Contents

Acknowledgements

Thanks go to the following people: for reading the text and constructive help Peter Husband; Peter Trott for photomicrographs; Peter Hamilton for my teaching and the fundal photographs, and Stanley Jablonski (Jablonski's Syndromes and Eponymic Diseases, Krieger Publishing, Florida, 1991) for solving the origins of eponyms!

Many of my friends generously gave me pictures that I lacked: Sir Richard Bayliss, **28**, **72**, **77**, **87**, **97**, **142**, **448**, **600**, **681**, **742-744**, **806**; Dr C D Calnan, **849**; Mr Anthony Catterall, **512**; Dr William E Clarke, **629**; Sir Anthony Dawson, **537**, **622**, **623**, **655**, **657**, **658**, **662**, **663**, **847**, **848**; Institute of Dermatology, **849**, **850**; Mr Frank G Ellis, **400**, **534**, **535**, **787**; Dr Peter Emerson, **790**; Dr R T D Emond, **333**; Mr Peter Hamilton, **238**, **252a-259d**; Dr Clive Harmer, **556**, **557**; Professor Janet Husband, **109**, **110**, **204**, **590**; Dr D G James, **62**; Sir Francis Avery Jones; **283**, **284**; Mr L W Kay, **317-319**; Professor Neil Macintyre, **240**, **241**; Dr Imry Sarkany, **68**, **69**, **79**, **98**, **808**; Dr Margaret Spittle, **316**, **553-556**; Mr Richard Staughton, **349**; Sir Rodney Sweetnam, **236**; Dr Peter Trott, **114**, **271**; Dr Alan Walker, **123**, **463**, **482**, **538**; Wellcome Trustees, **752**; Dr A Wisdom, **289**; Dr I Zamiri, **333**; Dr Kevin Zilkha, **65**, **187**, **188**, **194-196**, **514**.

Preface

Physical signs are like wild flowers, either chanced upon while you are out for a walk or sought with prior knowledge of their habitat. In medicine the student may detect physical signs as he scans the patient from face to hand and from head to trunk: the seasoned physician sees a physical sign and knows where to look for confirmation of its significance.

This collection of clinical photographs is an eclectic selection which broadly embraces general internal medicine. The pictures are arranged anatomically, rather than by diseases, because physical signs are seen topographically. Thus, pictures relating to one condition may be found in different parts of the book.

The photographs show the appearance of a physical sign as seen at the bedside, and include the minor as well as the obvious and gross. Sometimes, several pictures of the same condition are shown so that the characteristic features of the disease can be correlated.

Photographs of physical signs may sometimes be dull and repetitive. Problem pictures are more fun. Thus, where possible, the caption begins with the clinical context in which to frame your thoughts, then describes the picture in order to heighten your interest, draws attention to the detail and gives the highlighted diagnosis. Where appropriate, the causes, differential diagnoses and additional points to look for are mentioned.

The undergraduate will study a wide selection of short cases and a number of very common conditions are included. For both the undergraduate and the postgraduate the illustrations provide useful comparisons with photographs used in examinations.

The photographs were taken either at the bedside or in the consulting room and clinic. Electronic flash was used for most pictures, although the African photographs were taken in available light at an aperture of f1.8 and so have a very shallow depth of field.

Michael Zatouroff

To Diana

THE HEAD

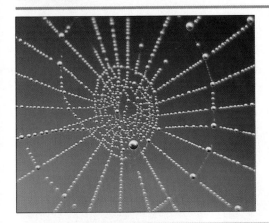

1 A spider's web. You see an empty spider's web—but look and think about the component parts. The dew drop is a convex lens. This will invert the image seen in the drop, yet the skyline is above and the earth below—so the picture is upside down. **Now** you see an upside-down spider's web and dew drops will never be the same! Just gazing is not enough. The brain must think about what the eyes see.

*YOU ONLY **SEE** WHAT YOU HAVE BEEN **TAUGHT** TO SEE.*

THE FACE

Figures **2–8** show normal people. These people are all 'healthy and uncomplaining'. They appear that way, but what do you observe in favour of this conclusion? Think about the component parts...*why are they all healthy?*

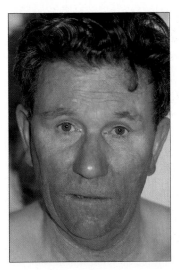

2 An outdoor worker. He's plethoric, no longer slim, and alert. Most of your reasons for health will be based on what you do *not* see. He isn't jaundiced, anaemic or cachexic—these features are absent. But health must also have positive signs that allow one to infer that it is present.

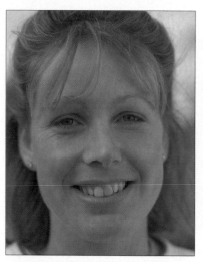

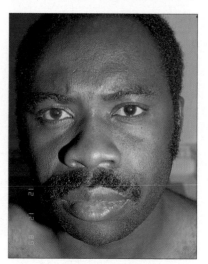

3 A young Caucasian equestrian stable manager. The most striking aspect is that she is happy. Mood is a positive sign when summing up appearance.

4 A West African academic. He is serious and well nourished with shiny black hair and a dense rich colour which would go greyer if he was anaemic.

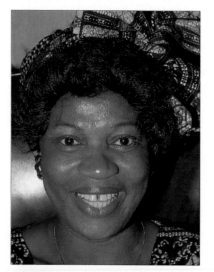

5 A West African senior nurse. The manner of presentation to the world will reflect how one feels. Taking care over appearance reflects priorities—and mood. The use of cosmetics should be a positive observation. They may not be used if her mind is preoccupied with other anxieties.

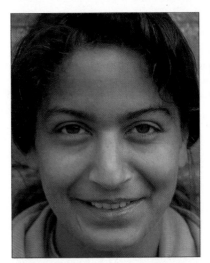

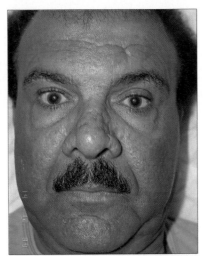

6 A south-east Asian dressage rider. A young woman whose family originated in the Indian subcontinent. She smiles. The brown skin may cause confusion if she becomes jaundiced or pale. Generally richness of colour is lost.

7 A middle-aged Middle Eastern retired businessman. He is well nourished, has pink mucous membranes, and has dyed his hair—the roots just show white at the hairline. He also has a corneal arcus, a scar on the left temple and a pitted skin whose distribution reflects smallpox as a child, all pertinent but irrelevant abnormalities which should be noted as they tell a great deal about his past.

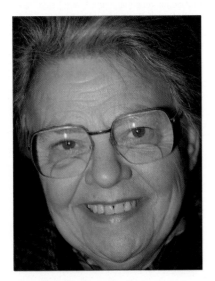

All these individuals are healthy. They fit into the range which you have learnt is normal and which you continually update and refine.

8 An elderly Caucasian clinical teacher. All ages have their appearance. Mood is critical and reflects symptoms. She is well groomed, nourished and presented. Presbyopia requires bifocal spectacles as near vision is necessary to read, work, knit and observe.

Colour changes in the skin

PALLOR

This is not synonymous with anaemia, and is altered by pigmentation or vaso-constriction as well as a fall in the haemoglobin level. It should be confirmed by comparing the skin with a normal capillary bed.

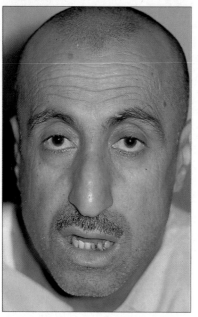

9 A pale man from Arabia. He complains of rectal bleeding. The skin is brown and he looks yellow. The lips are pale and he looks apathetic. *See* **10 and 11** for the appearance of his mouth.

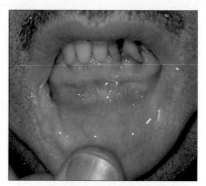

10 The buccal mucosa confirms the pallor (before transfusion) and contrasts with the examiner's nail bed. He smokes (notice his nicotine-stained teeth) and has periodontal disease leading to gum recession.

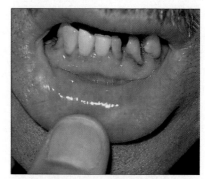

11 His buccal mucosa after blood transfusion.

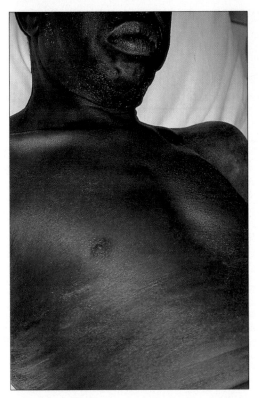

12 A pale black skin in a West African farmer. The skin looks grey, which is pallor. Nuances of colour are important in prompting such thoughts. A haemoglobin of 5 g/dl can be missed in active farmers with hookworm infestation when the anaemia has developed slowly. The skin shows recent weight loss because it falls in shallow folds. When the buccal mucosa is compared with the examiner's nail bed the contrast is clear (see **13**).

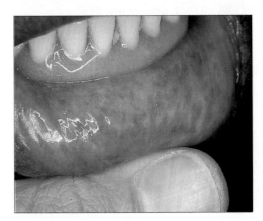

13 A pale West African. Buccal mucosa compared with a nail capillary bed.

5

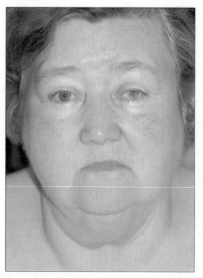

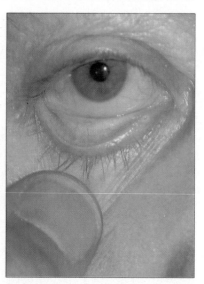

14 A Caucasian woman—pale but not anaemic. A malar flush with dilated superficial veins, a left corneal arcus, and a roundness of the face from obesity. The hair has been coloured. The haemoglobin is 14 g/dl and underlines the danger of using observed pallor as the sole index of anaemia.

15 Her conjunctiva looks pale compared to the examiner's nail bed!

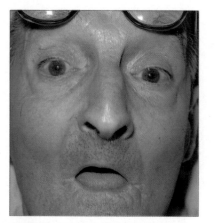

16 A pale man with angular stomatitis. Slight pallor of the lips, a tint of jaundice of the sclera and a smooth tongue. There is healed angular stomatitis, which is probably related to his habit of going without his dentures, allowing over-closure of the mouth and soreness at the corners of the mouth. He has a macrocytic anaemia.

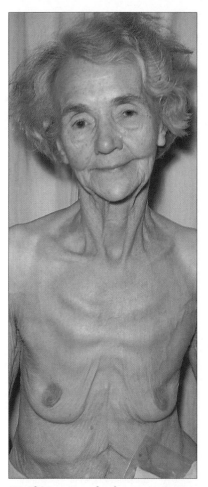

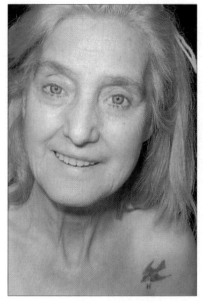

18 A woman of middle age.
The lips and face are pale, the hair prematurely grey and the eyes blue. There is pallor of the lower lid margin and a tattoo on the left shoulder, which may be associated with other viral diseases. The facies of **pernicious anaemia** are due to vitamin B_{12} deficiency.

17 This woman had a gastrectomy many years earlier. Pallor and weight loss are present. Her iron deficiency anaemia was ascribed to poor iron absorption and her diet. An error in this age group, for a colonic carcinoma is a common cause of occult blood loss in the elderly. The colonic carcinoma was found after her anaemia failed to respond. The stoma bag just shows in the left iliac fossa.

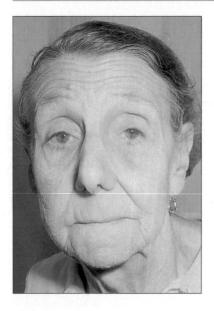

19 The facies of Pernicious anaemia. Facial pallor, blue eyes and grey hair. Remember to look for other organ associated autoimmune disease. A tingling of the hands may be present due to the neuropathy of vitamin B12 deficiency or may represent median nerve compression and coexisting autoimmune hypothyroidism.

HYPERPIGMENTATION

Hyperpigmentation may be due to friction or sunlight, race or disease (neuro-fibromatosis, melanomatosis, haemochromatosis, thyrotoxicosis, exogenous or endogenous excess adrenocorticotrophic hormone (ACTH)). It can be due to pigment deposition from bilirubin, carotene, drugs (clofazimine, minocycline and mepacrine), metals (lead, mercury and gold) or arsenic. It can also be found in association with malnutrition or pregnancy. Look for the surface application of cosmetics, perfumes and chemicals like silver nitrate, which may colour or sensitise to light.

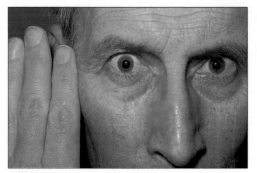

20 A grey man with mild diabetes, sparse secondary sexual hair and a large liver and spleen. When compared to the normal hand, his skin has a slate-grey colour associated with increased dermal melanin. **Haemochromatosis.** The joint involvement may show calcification in cartilage (*see* **21**).

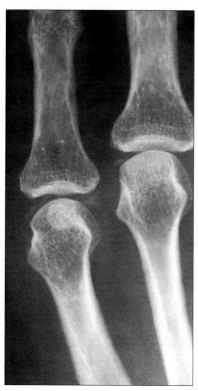

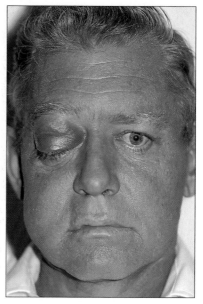

22 In this man, a melanoma of the thigh was removed 15 years earlier. He presented with a large liver and then became hyperpigmented due to disseminated **malignant melanomatosis**. Note the secondary melanoma of the orbit.

21 Chondrocalcinosis. The calcification in the articular cartilage is seen in the joint space of the metacarpo-phalangeal joint. It is found in degenerative joint disease, after trauma to cartilage, in pseudogout and gout, and in disordered copper metabolism(Wilson's disease – hepatolenticular degeneration), iron metabolism (haemochromatosis) and calcium metabolism (hyperparathyroidism). It is a feature of ochronosis (alcaptonuria) (*see* **264**).

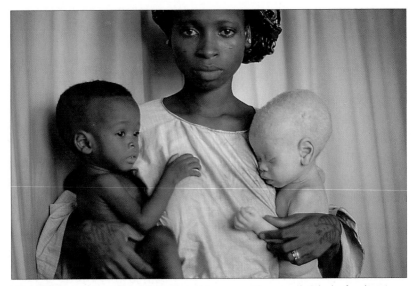

23 Albinism. Dizygotic twins in West Africa, one with a complete lack of melanin. This is due to a single pair of mutant genes leading to tyrosine deficiency and the ultimate failure of pigment formation in eye and skin. At least 10 types are known. There is an increased risk of skin cancer and defects in white cell function and haemostasis may occur. Impaired vision and nystagmus are common. Oculocutaneous albinism may be associated with loss of binocular vision from optic tract defects when all fibres cross to the opposite side.

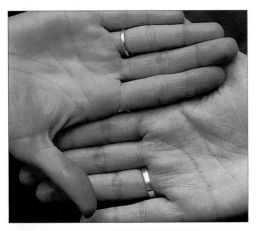

24 Carotenaemia. The mother (on the right) and her daughter (on the left). The yellow pigmentation is due to carotene. This young woman ate excess mangoes and carrots (up to 4 kilos daily in an attempt at weight reduction), although pawpaw and oranges are often the culprits. A yellow tint of the skin associated with high levels of betacarotene may also be seen in hypothyroidism due to a defect in enzyme conversion to vitamin A. It is also a feature of lipoproteinaemia.

DEPIGMENTATION

Depigmentation may be localised or widespread. Causes include infection (*see* leprosy, **855**, where the depigmentation, in contrast with vitiligo, is not total; yeast, *see* pityriasis versicolor, **43**) and failure of melanin production after inflammation.

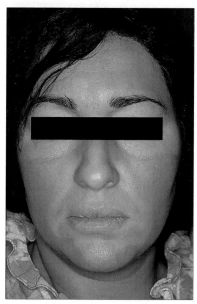

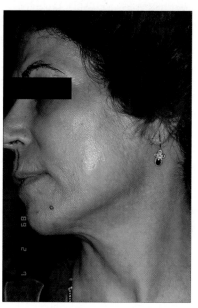

25 Vitiligo. Depigmentation around the eyes and mouth of an otherwise healthy woman. This is an autoimmune disease which may be associated with other coexisting organ specific autoimmune diseases (pernicious anaemia, hypothyroidism, Addison's[1] disease and diabetes should be considered). There is often a family history. There may be a curious symmetry which is without explanation, whilst the cosmetic problem is greatest in those who are heavily pigmented.

26 Adrenocortical insufficiency—Addison's disease. This may be due to primary adrenal destruction, usually autoimmune or less commonly as a result of tuberculosis or secondary to pituitary disease. Vitiligo may be present. The skin is hyperpigmented as if sun-tanned, though the colour is patchy.

---

[1] Sir Thomas Addison, English physician,1793–1860. Anaemia—disease of the suprarenal capsules. *Lond. Hosp. Gaz.*, 1849, **43**: 517–18.

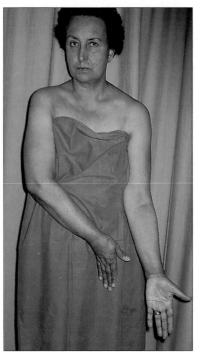

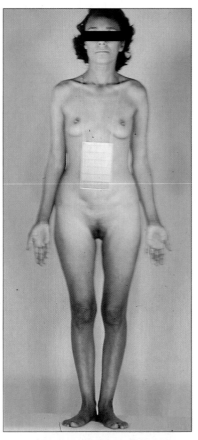

27 Excess endogenous adrenocorticotrophic hormone (ACTH)—Nelson's syndrome[2]. It is February and this Caucasian native of southeast England has *not* just come from sunny Spain. The apparent tan is not only over the face, exposed surfaces of the arms, hands and neckline, but also present in the palmar skin creases and under the bra strap. It is caused by excess ACTH and increased melanin production. This lady has had a bilateral adrenalectomy for adrenal hyperplasia, but has a pituitary adenoma secreting ACTH.

28 Adrenocortical insufficiency— Addison's disease. A gradual onset of tiredness led to this woman's consultation. There is a striking darkening of the exposed skin and around the vulva as well as palmar pigmentation. Compare this with racial and henna palmar pigmentation (*see* **364, 375**).

---

[2]Nelson DH (U.S.physician) *et al.* ACTH producing tumour of the pituitary gland. *N. Eng. J. Med.,* 1958, **259**:161–4.

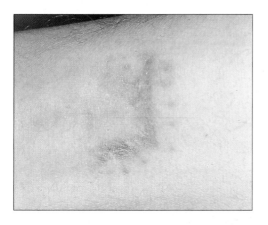

29 Addisonian pigmentation. Pigmentation may occur in surgical scars. Here the scar of an old varicose vein operation has pigmented. All scars should be examined. Darkening may occur over pressure areas and on the gums as well as on exposed parts of the body.

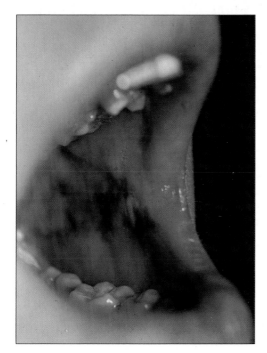

30 Addisonian pigmentation on the buccal mucosa. Pigmentation is seen on the inside of the cheek. This is significant in Caucasians, but may be a normal finding in dark-skinned races.

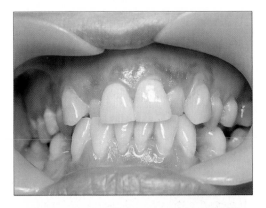

31 Addison's disease (gum pigmentation). This occurs on the gum away from the periodontal edge and must not be confused with normal racial pigmentation of the gums (see **32**).

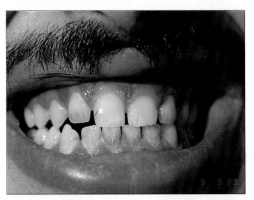

32 Normal racial pigmentation of the gums. Dark-skinned races have patchy pigmented areas in the mouth, which can confuse the inexperienced. This also shows brown nicotine-stained dental plaque.

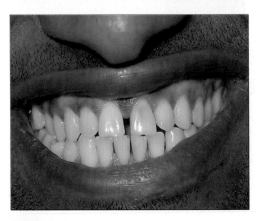

33 Gum tattooing. In Ethiopia and Sudan some women tattoo their gums to heighten the contrast with white teeth. Therapeutic tattooing may be used in the belief that it will strengthen loose teeth. This man's tooth was loosened by a blow. It is discoloured. The gum at the base was tattooed and with time, the tooth stopped rocking in its socket! One area of pigment looked incongruous, so alternate areas were tattooed.

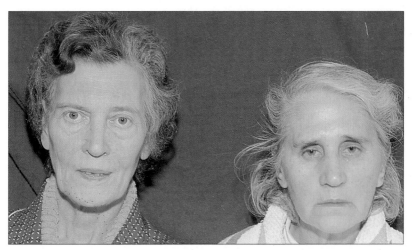

34 Jaundice of the face. Jaundice on the left is compared with a normal non-jaundiced appearance on the right. The yellow tint is best seen in the conjunctiva once the bilirubin is greater than 50 μmol/l or thrice the normal level. A white skin may also show the staining on unexposed areas. It is best seen in daylight and can be mimicked if the bedspread or clothes, such as the dressing gown on the right, reflect their colour, as well as by the effect of ageing on, or the deposition of fat in, the conjunctiva.

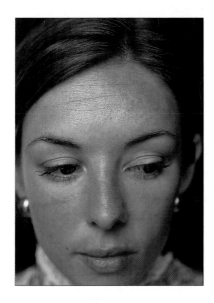

35 Melanosis or chloasma of the face. Pigmentation of the forehead or cheeks is common in females during pregnancy and in those taking the contraceptive pill. Pigmentation may also appear if perfumes are applied to sun-exposed areas and is common in darker-skinned people, especially in the Middle East.

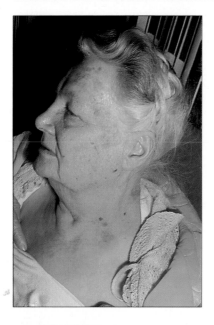

36 Senile hyperkeratosis. Brown raised keratotic patches occurring with age. This is a non-malignant condition and is common in the elderly. It should be differentiated from basal cell carcinoma between the hyperkeratotic areas. Solar lentigo—macular areas of brown pigmentation—may appear in the elderly and in those exposed to sunlight.

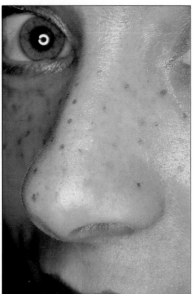

37 The ephelis or freckle. This is common in children and among the fair- or red-headed. It is a pale brown macule, usually about 2–3 mm in diameter with an ill-defined edge. Normal melanocytes produce more melanin in response to ultraviolet light. With increasing awareness of the dangers of sun exposure they may even be painted on! Freckles fade in the winter in contrast to a **lentigo**, which persists in the absence of ultraviolet light and is a feature of Peutz–Jeghers syndrome and increasing age. A **lentigo** may darken in pregnancy and in Addison's disease (adrenocortical insufficiency).

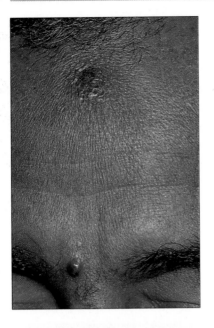

38 Prayer callus in a Muslim cleric. Repeated friction leads to thickening of the skin, pigmentation and callus. The frequency and force will produce varying degrees of discoloration. This cleric has a marked callus compared to that of the devout lay Muslim (*see* **39**).

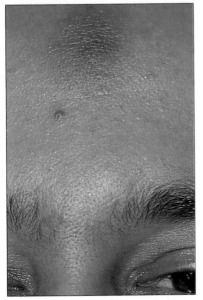

39 Prayer callus in a devout lay Muslim diabetic. The appreciation of the cause will aid the physician in planning diet and dose schedules, which may require modification at times of fasting.

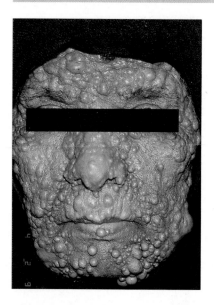

40 von Recklinghausen's disease (Neurofibromatosis[3] (NF) type I face).

Patchy pigmentation due to café au lait spots may be marked, but is overshadowed by the presence of multiple 2–5 mm nodular neurofibromas on the skin. This autosomal dominant condition may exhibit incomplete penetrance and there may be little to see on the skin except a single café au lait spot and sparse nodules. The eyes should be examined for iris hamartomas (*see* **239**). In von Recklinghausen's[3] original description the patient had café au lait spots and neurofibromas and gut lesions leading to intussusception.

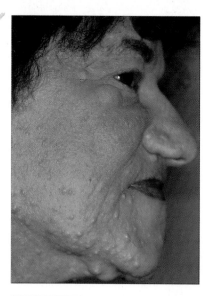

41 Neurofibromatosis type 1 Caucasian face.

The nodules vary from 3–10 mm in size and are less raised. None were present before the age of 10 years.

[3] Recklinghausen, F.D. von. German pathologist, 1833–1910. *Über die multiplen Fibrome der Haut und ihre Beziehungen zu den Neuromen.* Berlin, A. Hirschwald, 1882.

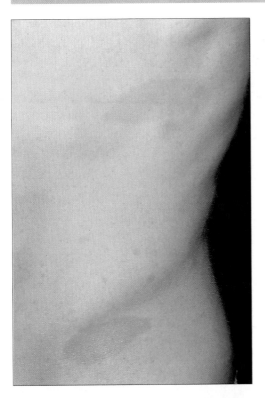

42 Neurofibromatosis (NF) type 1 café au lait spots.
Café au lait spots vary in size and continue to appear throughout life. Usually there are more than six. Freckles may be seen in the axilla. This is type NF 1, which is carried by a defective gene on chromosome 17, in contrast to type 2, which is carried on chromosome 22 (so-called central NF in which cutaneous manifestations may be sparse and iris nodules absent, but there are associated bilateral acoustic neuromas).

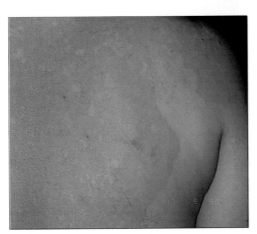

43 Pityriasis versicolor.
A superficial resemblance to café au lait spots and usually appearing on the upper trunk. This is not to be confused with the hypopigmentation of tuberculoid leprosy (see **855**) or vitiligo (see **25**). It is caused by the superficial fungus *Malassezia furfur*. It is common, becomes more obvious if sun-tanned, varies in colour and may have a characteristic, bran scale-like appearance, which is reflected in its name.

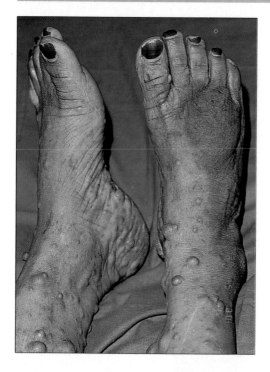

44 Neurofibromatosis type 1 plexiform neuroma on the foot. The presence of a plexiform neurofibroma is characteristic. The flat raised area over the dorsum of the right foot also shows a coffee coloured spot. If café au lait spots, iris nodules and neuromas have not appeared by the late teens then the chance of inheritance is low.[4] Henna had been applied to the toes about three weeks earlier. Note the rate of nail growth.

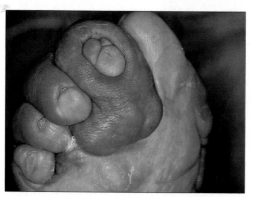

45 Neurofibromatosis type 1 plexiform neuroma on the toe. This may encircle a limb or a digit and earn the description *elephantiasis neurofibromatosa*.

---

[4]A full description of this fascinating disease is given in two articles: Case records of the Massachusetts General Hospital. *N. Eng. J. Med.*, 1989, **320 (15)**: 996–1004, which covers all the associations with neuroendocrine tumours; and Lubs *et al.* Lisch nodules in Neurofibromatosis Type 1. *N. Eng. J. Med.*, 1991, **324 (18)**: 1264–6, which discusses iris hamartomas and their significance.

THE RED FACE AND RED SPOTS/BLEMISHES/MARKS

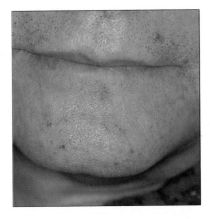

46 Hereditary haemorrhagic telangiectasia (Osler[5]–Weber[6]–Rendu[7] disease[8]).
This man with recurrent gastrointestinal bleeding was finally diagnosed when he shaved off his moustache and the telangiectases around the mouth were noted. Focal dilation of postcapillary venules are seen around the lips, on the buccal mucosa, and on the cheeks. In the interim he had had a gastrectomy, developed malabsorption and tuberculosis! Vascular abnormalities of the skin, nose, gut, lung and brain may bleed, and a high output state may develop.

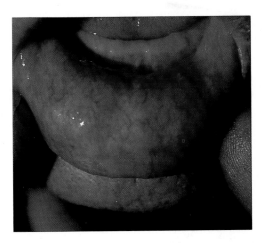

47 Hereditary haemorrhagic telangiectasia (lips).
Dilation of postcapillary venules is seen around the lips.

[5]Sir William Osler, Canadian physician, 1849–1919. Osler W. On multiple hereditary telangiectases with recurrent haemorrhage. *Q. J. Med.(Oxford)*, 1907, **1**: 53–8.
[6]Frederick Parkes Weber, British physician, 1863–1962. Weber PF. A note on cutaneous telangiectases and their aetiology. Comparison with the aetiology of haemorrhoids and ordinary varicose veins. *Edinburgh Med. J.*, 1904, 346–9.
[7]Henri Jules Louis Marie Rendu, French physician, 1844–1902. Rendu H. Epistaxis répetées chez un sujet porteur de petits angiomes cutanés et muqueux. *Bull. Spc. Méd. Hôp. (Paris)*, 1896, **13**: 731–3.
[8]Guttmacher *et al.* Hereditary haemorrhagic telangiectasia review article. *N. Eng. J. Med.*, 1995, **333** (**14**): 918–24.

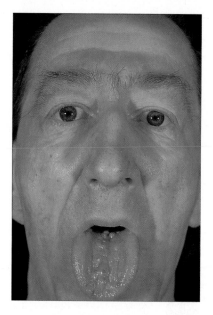

48 Hereditary haemorrhagic telangiectasia. Dilation of venules is seen on the face. Arteriovenous (a/v) malformations such as those on the tongue may lack capillaries and consist of direct a/v connections. Approximately 5–10% of patients have pulmonary a/v malformations, and symptomatic shunting and cyanosis may occur. Finger nail clubbing may be a feature.

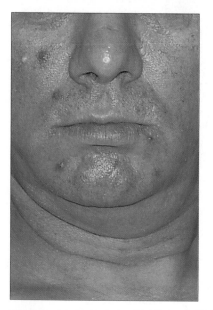

49 Spider naevi on the face. A tint of jaundice in the conjunctiva and extensive spider naevi due to chronic liver disease. The central feeding vessel and the radiating capillaries are seen. Pressure on the centre produces blanching. Distributed on the upper trunk and face, they occur in pregnancy when they may disappear within hours of delivery, and may occur in normal people, enlarging with the menses. They also occur in association with high output states and in liver disease.

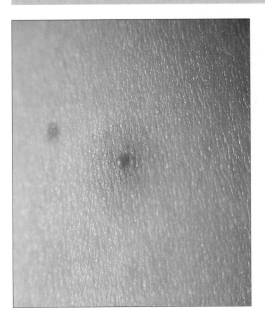

50 Spider naevus.
Pressure on the centre results in blanching, and release demonstrates the radiating capillary network.

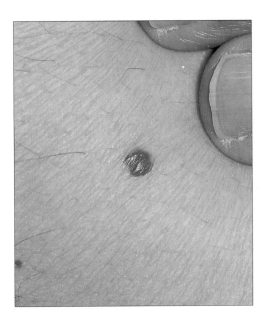

51 Cherry angiomas (*syn.* Campbell de Morgan spots).
These are common with increasing age and usually occur on the trunk. Histologically they are angiokeratomas. They may vary in number and may disappear. Similar spots may occur on the scrotum.

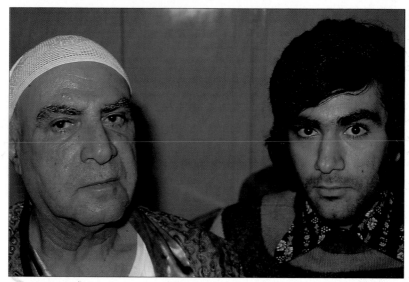

52 Middle Eastern polycythaemic man and his normal son. Facial plethora may be obvious, but is easily overlooked if the skin is pigmented. Conjunctival suffusion is present. Dark skins will look darker with the increase in background red.

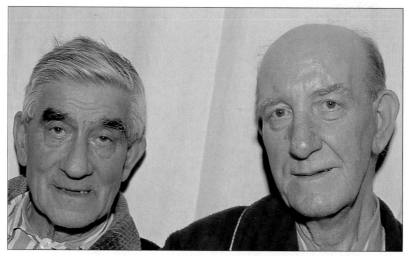

53 Caucasian polycythaemic man and control. Conjunctival suffusion and plethora must not be ascribed to health. The veins in the fundi may look black.

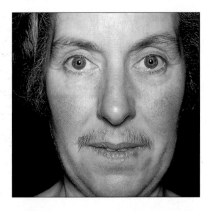

54 Mitral malar flush—mitral stenosis. Redness of the cheeks may be seen in health and in outdoor workers and reflect the effect of cold. In those on steroid therapy it may be due to thinning of the skin. Its presence in mitral stenosis and the description of mitral facies is now rare; in this context it may represent poor cardiac output, but its origin remains unclear.

FACIAL FLUSHING

Facial flushing may be emotional, hormonal, occur at the menopause, or be induced by alcoholic drinks or in diabetics by chlorpropamide. It may also be seen in disease:

- In the carcinoid syndrome with tachycardia, wheeze or loose stools. Facial flushing may become fixed.
- In systemic mastocytosis, facial flushing may be associated with a headache.
- Facial flushing is a manifestation of phaeochromocytomas and neuro-ganglionomas secreting adrenaline and noradrenaline precursors.
- In rosacea, flushing may be associated with food and alcohol.

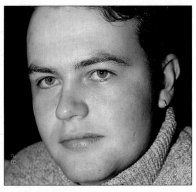

55 Facial flush before alcohol.

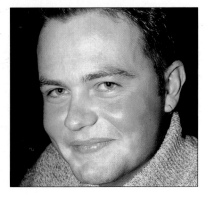

56 Alcohol flush after a bottle of Claret. It may reveal subclinical carcinoid syndrome or mastocytosis, but probably reflects the metabolic consequences of handling acetaldehyde and other metabolites. Alcohol-induced flushing occurs in rosacea.

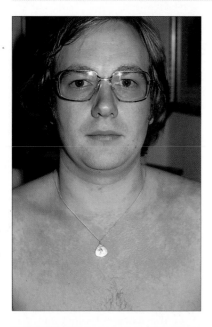

57 Blush rash. The anxiety associated with physical examination often precipitates a pink mottling of the upper trunk, which gradually subsides as the patient relaxes.

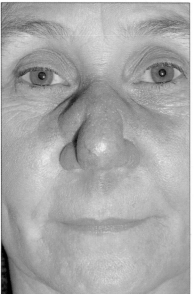

58 Lupus pernio nose. The characteristic blue purple colour of chronic sarcoid infiltrating the skin. Dilated pilosebaceous follicles are visible and pustulation is absent. It may be associated with facial palsy and lymphoedema of the lips—the Melkersson–Rosenthal syndrome. A variant with a coloured border and atrophic centre must be differentiated from tuberculoid leprosy (*see* **855**).

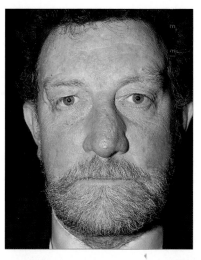

59 Malar rash (lupus pernio). The rash overlies the cheeks and forehead, there is no pustulation (*see* rosacea, **70**), but the area about the eyes is spared. The purple–red colour is characteristic. It must not be confused with systemic lupus.

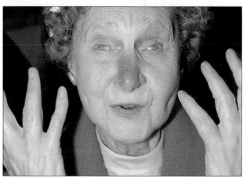

60 Lupus pernio (blindness and dactylitis). This is more common in women, and may be associated with bone cysts, which are reflected in swelling of the digits, and uveitis, which has led to blindness.

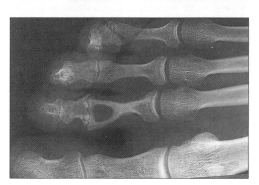

61 Radiograph of bone cysts in the toes.

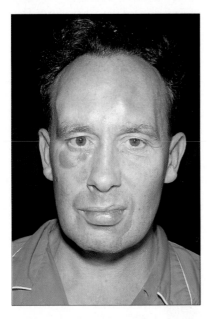

62 The Melkersson–Rosenthal[9] syndrome. Features include facial palsy, lymphoedema of the lips and an enlarged tongue. There may be associated cutaneous granulomas. Note the lupus pernio of the cheek, right-sided facial palsy and large swollen lips. Small skin creases around the eye are lost and the right side of the mouth droops slightly compared with the left.

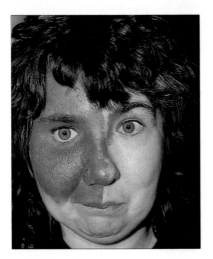

63 Sturge–Weber syndrome.[10] A cavernous haemangioma is confined to the territory of the ophthalmic and maxillary branches of the trigeminal nerve. There is a contralateral hemiplegia due to the ipsilateral haemangioma overlying the right motor cortex (tramline calcification of the vessels may be seen on the radiograph), which also leads to contralateral epileptic fits. The pain of associated absolute glaucoma led to enucleation of the eye. The glass eye has a perfectly white sclera and would be noticed if looked for!

[9] Melkersson, Ernst Gustav, Swedish physician, 1892–1932. Rosenthal, Curt, German physician.
[10] Described by William Allen Sturge, 1850–1919, in 1879, and by Frederick Parkes Weber, 1863–1962, in 1922.

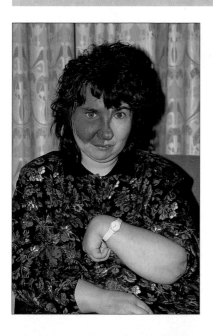

64 Sturge–Weber syndrome hemiplegic posture. The adducted arm, flexed and with a clenched fist, is smaller than the left. This woman always bought dresses with over-long sleeves to hide the contracture.

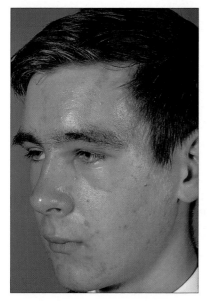

65 Mild Sturge–Weber syndrome. A capillary naevus is present over the ophthalmic branch of the trigeminal nerve. Acne may indicate that phenytoin is being prescribed for epilepsy.

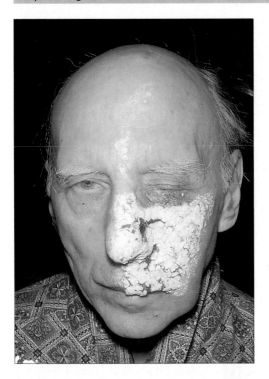

66 Herpes zoster of the maxillary branch of the fifth cranial nerve. This shows a dramatic appearance confined to the territory of the maxillary branch of the trigeminal nerve due to calamine lotion. Patients commonly apply substances to the skin, which may confuse the inexperienced. The vesicles extend up between the eyebrows along the zygomatic temporal branch of the zygomatic nerve, a branch of the maxillary division of the the fifth nerve having a variable temporal distribution.

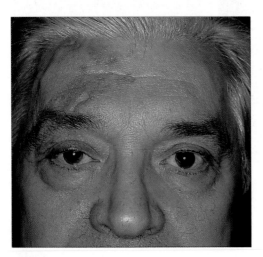

67 Healed herpes zoster of the ophthalmic branch of the fifth cranial nerve. Scarring in the distribution of the ophthalmic branch extends from the hair line to the vertex. Ophthalmic herpes may be associated with corneal ulceration. Herpes zoster affecting the geniculate ganglion may be associated with facial palsy and a rash in the ear (see **277**).

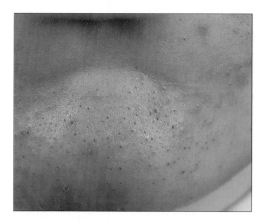

68 Acne vulgaris. This is characterised by chronic inflammation of the pilosebaceous unit. The skin is shiny due to increased sebum production, and ductal hypercornification leads to blackhead or comedone production.

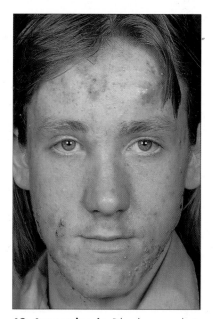

69 Acne vulgaris. Pilosebaceous duct blockage leads to cyst formation and inflammation.

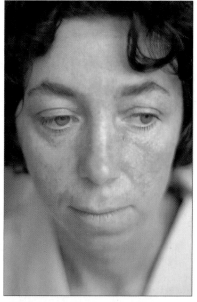

70 Rosacea. This is characterised by flushing, redness and telangiectasia over the cheeks and nasal bridge, sparing the eyes. Episodes of acneform pustulation and lymphoedema may lead to rhinophyma. Conjunctivitis is common and unexplained.

SYSTEMIC SCLEROSIS

Features of systemic sclerosis include extensive telangiectasia and a tightening of the skin, which may become shiny and lead to a pursed mouth appearance. Tautness of the skin around the mouth and neck may limit movement. The vertical lines around the mouth are prominent. Dilated vessels are also seen over the cheeks and in the hands, where the skin is taut and inelastic. Raynaud's phenomenon is common. Dilated facial capillaries are echoed by the periungual erythema of dilated capillary loops. This is also seen in dermatomyositis and systemic lupus erythematosus.

Scleroderma or localised morphoea is a localised sclerosis of the skin and may occur in systemic lupus erythematosus and dermatomyositis and as a cutaneous manifestation of systemic sclerosis. When confined to the skin alone it is termed morphoea.

The sabre cut (*en coup de sabre*) is linear morphoea. The name reflects the dramatic depression that may occur and lead to facial asymmetry. Heterochromia of the iris may also be a feature.

It is helpful to remember that skin changes on a white skin will look different on a dark one. Red rashes look black, and mauve or purple may appear darker.

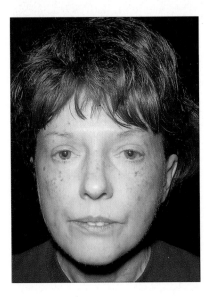

71 Systemic sclerosis. There are extensive telangiectases and a tightening of the skin, which may become shiny and lead to a pursed mouth appearance.

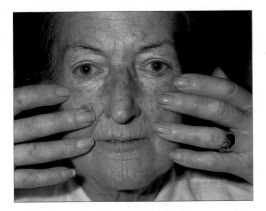

72 Systemic sclerosis. The vertical lines around the mouth are prominent. Dilated vessels over the cheeks are also seen in the hands, where the skin is taut and inelastic. Raynaud's phenomenon is common.

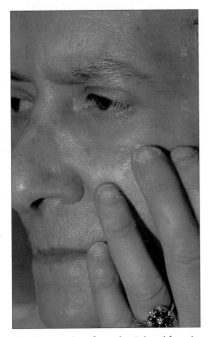

73 Systemic sclerosis. Dilated facial capillaries are echoed by the periungual erythema of dilated capillary loops. These are also a feature of dermatomyositis and systemic lupus erythematosus.

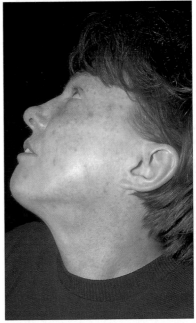

74 Systemic sclerosis. Tautness of the skin around the mouth and neck may limit movement.

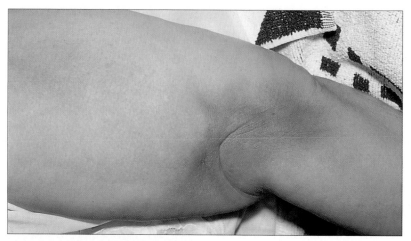

75 Scleroderma (localised morphoea). Localised sclerosis of the skin may occur in systemic lupus erythematosus and dermatomyositis, and as a cutaneous manifestation of systemic sclerosis. When confined to the skin alone it is termed morphoea. A circumscribed plaque is present on the arm with atrophy of the subcutaneous tissue and tethering of the skin.

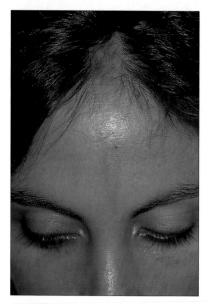

76 The sabre cut or *en coup de sabre* (linear morphoea). This lady wore a thick fringe to cover the linear depression, which passes up into her hair line producing linear alopecia. The name reflects the dramatic depression that may occur and lead to facial asymmetry. Heterochromia of the iris may be a feature.

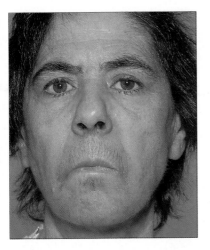

77 Dermatomyositis. The heliotrope[11] erythema around the eyes is characteristic, and may be associated with changes on the skin of the hands (*see* **380**). In the older patient there is an increased frequency of malignancy.

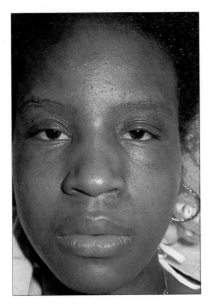

78 Dermatomyositis. This lady first noticed weakness when raising her arms to do her hair and then had difficulty in climbing stairs due to a severe proximal muscle weakness. On a pigmented skin the heliotrope colour becomes darker and is much more like bilateral bruising. The clinical context changes the differential diagnosis. If she was seen in a casualty department the first thought would be trauma. Note the pigmentation around the nose, which is also seen on the hands over the knuckles (*see* **380**).

---

[11]The word is rarely used in any other context except by gardeners, fashion writers or perfumers. To describe the purple colour by reference to a shrub, which turns its petals towards the sun and which few doctors would recognise, is frustrating. A student of Greek might think that it was due to sun worship.

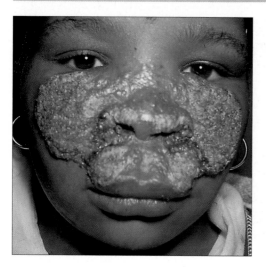

79 Lupus vulgaris (tuberculosis) of the face. Exuberant hypertrophic ulceration spreading over the nose and malar area. Lupus[12] vulgaris (*vulgar* = common) is due to tuberculosis, which may 'eat as a wolf'; lupus pernio (*see* **58/59**) is the 'sarcoid wolf'; and lupus erythematosus (*see* **85**) is the 'red wolf'.

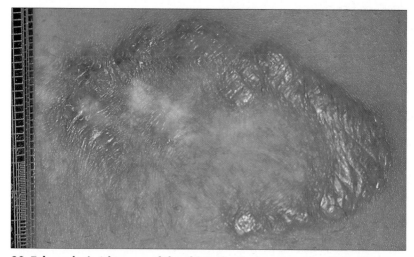

80 Tuberculosis (close-up of the skin). The classic appearance of cutaneous tuberculosis. A plaque made up of 'apple jelly' nodules with an area of central scarring.

---

[12]Lupus (Latin, a wolf).

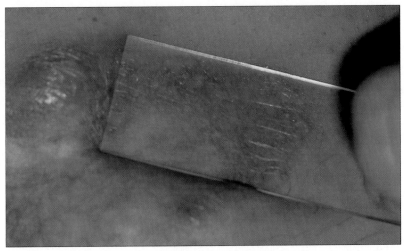

81 Tuberculosis (close-up of the skin as 'apple jelly'). When covered with a slide, the skin exhibits the typical 'apple jelly' appearance.

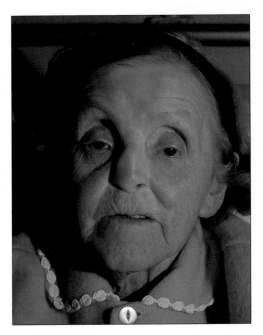

82 Lupus vulgaris (facial destruction). This may progress to scarring and destruction of cartilage. Secondary basal cell carcinoma may develop and be mistaken for a relapse.

THE MALAR RASH

The distribution of the malar rash over the cheeks and bridge of the nose may reflect the effect of the weather. This is the part of the face most prone to sunburn as well as to cold. Conditions associated with photosensitivity, whether drug induced, related to autoimmune disease or the application of perfume and cosmetics, may be associated with malar rashes. If the rash is labelled as a 'butterfly rash' because of its shape, the diagnosis is limited to lupus erythematosus.

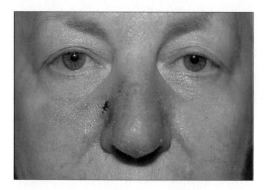

83 Systemic lupus erythematosus. A winter holiday to the Valley of the Kings in Egypt was cut short due to a fever, arthralgia and a rash on the face and legs. The malar distribution reflects those parts that catch the sun. There is a skin biopsy suture. Erythema on light-exposed areas occurs in up to 80% of patients at some stage and may be the presenting feature.

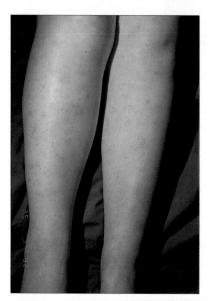

84 Systemic lupus erythematosus. The rash, provoked by sunlight, is seen on the legs, and the line produced by the calf-length skirt is seen.

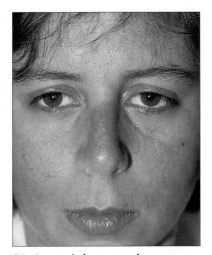

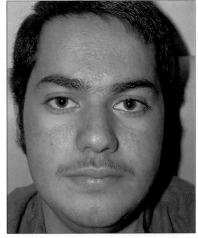

85 Systemic lupus erythematosus (malar rash). This young Gibraltarian girl was a keen sun worshipper and her illness began in early summer. Exposed areas of her face are affected.

86 Systemic lupus erythematosus (malar rash). This man presented with joint pain and oedema; he has a bat's wing malar erythema and forehead rash with maculopapular changes over his cheeks.

87 Systemic lupus erythematosus. The rash extends into the neckline and there is oedema of the lips.

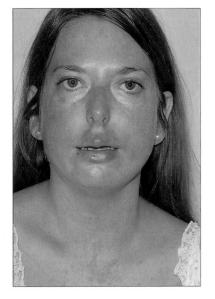

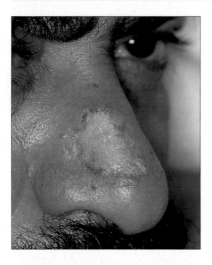

88 Chronic discoid lupus erythematosus. Well-defined scaly reddish patches, which heal with scarring. It is benign and most often involves the head. This discoid discrete active area on the nose has an active margin and atrophic centre.

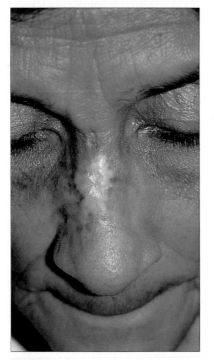

89 Chronic discoid lupus erythematosus. Healing is followed by central atrophic scarring.

HAIR

Hair loss

Hair growth is intermittent and depends on the cyclical activity of the hair follicle. Follicular activity is divided into three phases: **Anagen**, a period of growth; **Catagen**, a transitional period, when the hair undergoes involution, the root becomes clubbed and the hair is shed; and a resting phase, **Telogen**, after which the **A.C.T.** cycle begins again. Each follicle cycles independently of its neighbours. At any time 1% of hair follicles may be in catagen. Stress and systemic disease may precipitate a higher proportion into catagen simultaneously and accounts for the shedding (telogen effluvium) that may occur in these situations. The progress to catagen may be slowed at the end of pregnancy by hormonal changes and be responsible for loss in the four to six months after delivery, when the number of follicles in telogen may be increased. Androgen dependent hair loss may reflect the presence of more available androgen. Thyroid hormones affect growth and their lack leads to thinning seen in hypothyroidism. Hair loss may be traumatic, due to scarring or associated with scalp disorders.

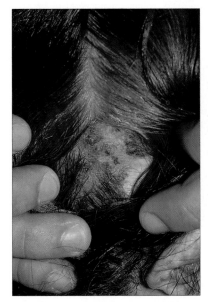

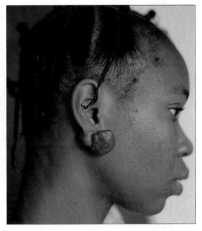

91 Traction alopecia. In Nigeria the hair may be plaited very tightly and lead to hair loss from mechanical damage. A similar hair loss at the temples may occur if a pony tail is habitually pulled very tight. A keloid scar has developed on the ear lobe—often this occurs on one side only and may reflect the direction of initial perforation—why?

90 Chronic discoid lupus on the scalp. Follicular plugging leads to the warty appearance. Healing with fibrous scarring leads to permanent hair loss.

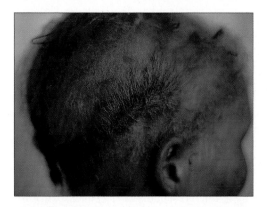

92 Malnutrition and a change in hair colour. This woman with diarrhoea has pale brown hair, which was black—traction alopecia is also present. Small bowel resection, ulcerative colitis and protein calorie malnutrition may cause black hair to become brown or reddish, and brown hair lighter still. If intermittent, then banding of colour may occur—*signe de la bandera.*

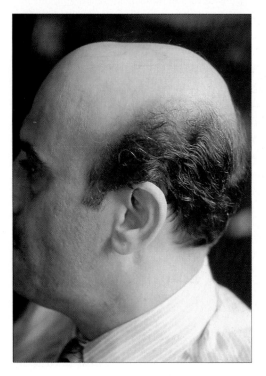

93 Androgenetic or male pattern balding (Hamilton grade VIII[13]). This is a manifestation of sexual maturity and is also seen in apes. Postmenopausal women may show a tendency to male pattern loss, hence the widow's peak.

---

[13]Hamilton JB. Patterned long hair in man; types and incidence. *Ann. NY. Acad. Sci.,* 1951, **53**: 708-14. Staging I–VIII of male pattern balding.

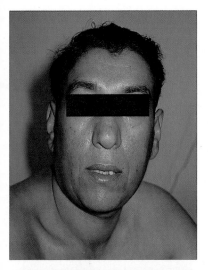

94 Widow's peak in male. This man has diminished hair growth on the trunk, limbs and beard area. He also had small testes and gynaecomastia. Klinefelter's syndrome (47 chromosomes, XXY sex chromosome complement) occurs in one in 600 male births and manifests at puberty with a failure to produce adult levels of testosterone and minimal development of secondary sexual characteristics.

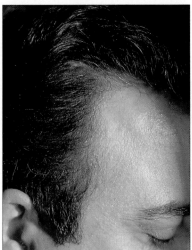

95 Frontal recession (grade III) and psoriasis in the scalp. Common scalp psoriasis is not a frequent cause of hair loss, and a seborrhoeic-like form may be seen.

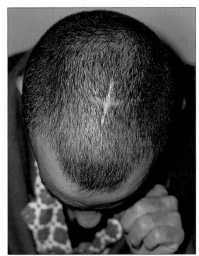

96 Frontal recession and cautery on scalp. Androgenetic-pattern baldness with temporal recession. This man had a severe headache and was found to have a meningioma. The cautery mark, from infancy, overlay the tumour—fortuitously, *x marked the spot!*

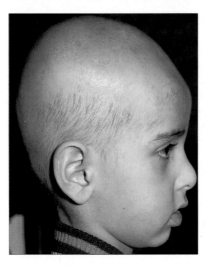

97 Diffuse alopecia secondary to irradiation. He has had low dose X-ray irradiation to the scalp as an outdated treatment for ring worm.

Chronic diffuse alopecia

This may be androgenetic or related to the hormonal changes of pregnancy or hypothyroidism. It can follow stress or illness—telogen effluvium—when much of the mosaic is precipitated into catagen, as well as by nutritional deficiency, chemical agents, cytotoxic drugs and external irradiation.

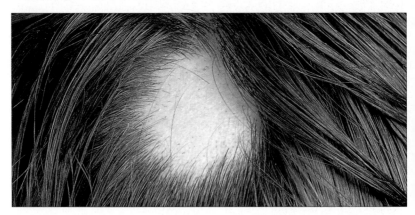

98 Alopecia areata of the scalp. This is a common problem. A patch of hair enters premature telogen. This may be local or total. The bald area may show broken short hairs—'exclamation mark hairs' due to weakening of the shaft seen at the margin. Nail changes including pitting, growth arrest lines and total loss may be seen. Regrowth may occur.

THE COARSENED FACE

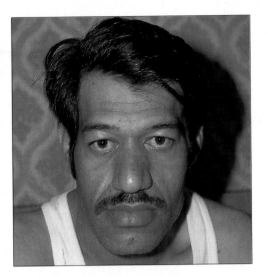

99 Acromegaly—the effect of excess growth hormone. This man felt the hot weather and sweated excessively. His features have become overemphasised and their delicacy is lost. He has a very prominent mandible and glabellar ridges, large lips and nose and a dramatic overbite, which all developed insidiously and are best appreciated by examining old photographs of the patient. The blurring of features with an increase in soft tissue may go unnoticed, with presentation related to intracranial pressure effects or an endocrine complication.

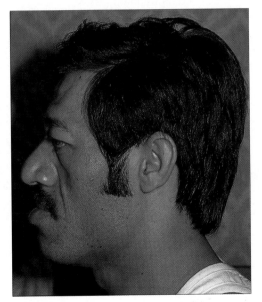

100 Acromegaly (side view). He spent his day in his vest because of his intolerance to central heating!

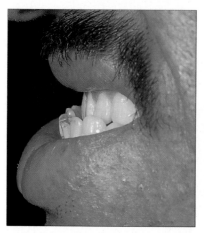

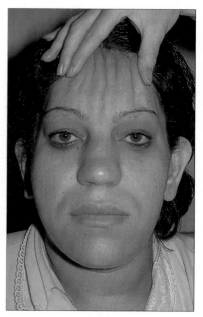

101 Acromegaly lantern jaw and big lips. An increase in the mandible leads to the prognathic jaw and overbite. An increase in tissue produces the big fleshy lips and the skin is greasy. This man's moustache is fashion, but a beard may reflect inner embarrassment and an attempt at camouflage.

102 Acromegaly showing an increase in soft tissue on the forehead. The classic complaint is the need to increase hat size. The reduplicated skin falls into corrugations and reflects the increase in soft tissue volume.

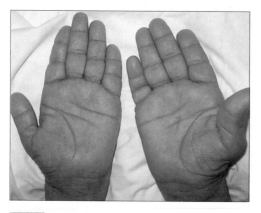

103 Acromegaly (hand). This lady complained of paraesthesiae of the hands at night and myalgia. She has an increase in the soft tissue and wasting of the thenar muscles. Abductor pollicis brevis wasting is obvious and suggests carpal tunnel compression of the median nerve. The causes of carpal tunnel syndrome must be reviewed or the diagnosis will be missed (*see* **page 409**).

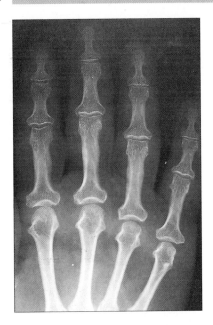

104 Acromegaly (radiograph of the hand). The increase in hand size and the carpal tunnel syndrome are related to the increase in soft tissue as well as to bony overgrowth, which is seen as tufting of the phalanges and broadening of the shaft. The increase in shoe size is due to broadening of the foot due to the increase in soft tissue. Joint symptoms must not be ascribed to simple ubiquitous degenerative joint disease.

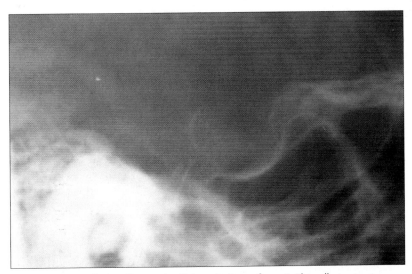

105 Acromegaly (radiograph of the pituitary fossa). The sella turcica is ballooned due to the pituitary adenoma.

BIG SKULL—HEAD

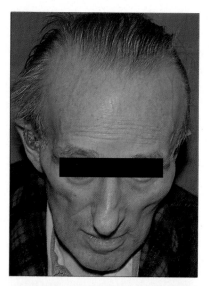

106 Paget's[14] disease of the skull (osteitis deformans). The increase in head size is due to expansion of bone and leads to diploic, rather than soft tissue, widening of the skull and an increase in skull diameter, leading to bossing. The auditory nerve may be compressed causing deafness. Note the hearing aid for the right ear.

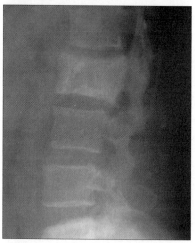

107 Paget's disease (radiograph of the lumbar spine).[15] This white vertebra differs from a metastasis because the change involves the whole vertebral body, with prominent horizontal trabeculae adjacent to the endplate leading to a box-like shape. It is soft and therefore may be squeezed out, in contrast to the wedging and collapse of infection and malignancy. The bone becomes denser and expands. Here the lumbar vertebra is wider and taller than its neighbours and this causes compression when a nerve passes through a bony foramen. In the skull this produces the changes seen in **106**.

[14]Sir James Paget, surgeon, 1814–1899; described in 1877.
[15]Harinck HIJ *et al.* Relationship between signs and symptoms in Paget's disease of bone—backache and deafness predominate. *Quart. J. Med.*, 1986, **58**:133–51.

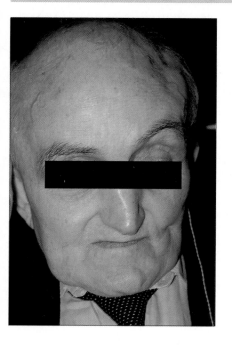

108 Paget's disease.
There is expansion of the skull
with irregularity. Note the
1960's National Health
Service hearing aid.

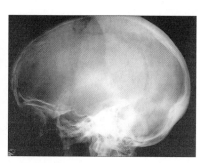

**109 Skull radiograph showing
osteoporosis circumscripta in
Paget's disease.** In the skull the two
stages of expansion and lysis may coexist.
Large areas of lysis, which are well
defined and are areas of great activity,
may be seen and are reflected in the bone
scan shown in **110** of an affected skull.

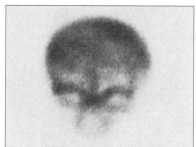

110 Bone scan of skull. Frontal view
showing osteoporosis circumscripta in
Paget's disease.

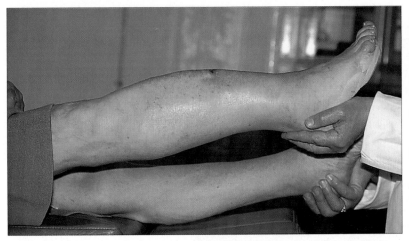

111 Paget's disease showing bowing of the tibia and enlargement of bone. The generalised bone softening results in bending of the right tibia, which typically bows forward. The soft bone bends and is wider and warmer than the left tibia. Basilar invagination may occur in the skull.

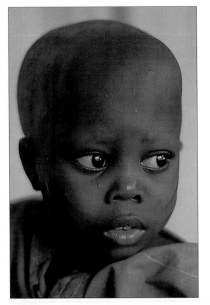

112 Sickle cell anaemia and skull bossing. This boy is pale and his conjunctivae are yellow. His skull vault has expanded. He has tribal scars on his cheeks. Bossing of the skull is due to extramedullary haematopoiesis, which causes skull expansion. This is a feature of untreated thalassaemia and sickle cell disease.

THE SCALP

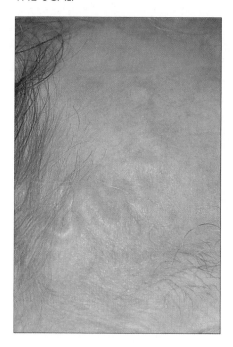

113 The prominent temporal artery—temporal arteritis. This Arabian woman's son, aged 45 years, was still single. 'Who will look after him if I die?—and I am so worried about Saddam Hussein' she said. Her severe temporal headache and aching shoulders were ascribed to stress. The artery is not particularly prominent and tenderness may be difficult to elicit. A finger on the artery and one on either side may allow the differential application of pressure and clarification of the symptom of pain. The erythrocyte sedimentation rate was 100 mm/hr.

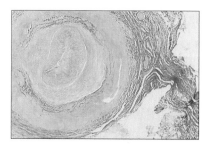

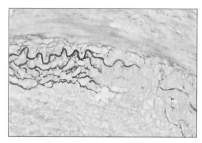

114 Temporal arteritis (histology). Transverse sections of the temporal artery show fibrous intimal proliferation obliterating the lumen and transmural granulomatous infiltration with partial destruction of the elastic laminae.

FAT (SWOLLEN/ENLARGED) FACE

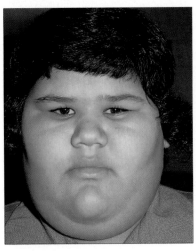

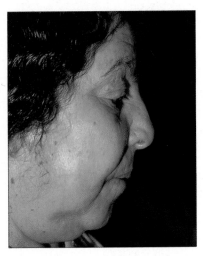

115 Fat face—body mass index (BMI) 43 kg/m². This 12-year-old boy was unable to see people standing next to him because of the severe obesity limiting his peripheral vision. He had no endocrine dysfunction. His height is 1.57 m and weight 106 kg. BMI = height in m² divided by weight in kg; normal is 20–25.

116 Fat face in middle age. This lady is moderately obese with a BMI of 30. She has apparently puffy facies and loss of lateral eye brow hair, but in conversation she is bright and jolly with brisk reflexes. Her thyroid function is normal.

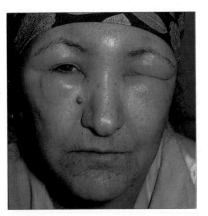

117 Facial oedema—nephritic facies. Variable, often non-pitting, oedema may be a feature of the acute nephritic syndrome when the puffiness affects the lax periorbital tissues. The appearance is the same, whether due to sodium retention, hypoalbuminaemia, protein malnutrition, local exudation, angioedema, urticaria, or allergy to insect bites or drugs.

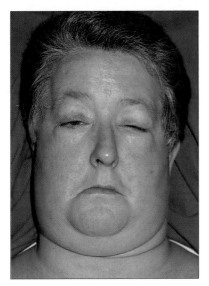

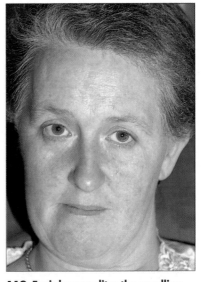

**118 Facial swelling—
subcutaneous emphysema.** This lady
developed sudden dramatic facial swelling
after coughing violently. A noise was
heard in time with the heart beat.

**119 Facial normality: the swelling
subsided over the next four days.**
Mediastinal emphysema with tracking of air
may occur with straining in labour, severe
coughing, in asthma or in divers on a rapid
uncontrolled ascent. Trauma and oesoph-
ageal rupture must be excluded. Hamman's
sign[16] is a noise in time with the heart
beating against air in the tissues.

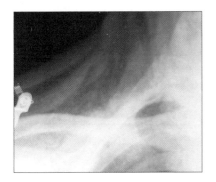

**120 Radiograph showing
subcutaneous emphysema.** The
subcutaneous air can be seen above the
clavicle to the right of the electrocardiogram electrode. On the chest radiograph,
mediastinal air may be seen as a line
adjacent to the cardiac border and must
be differentiated from lung cysts and a
pneumothorax.

[16]Louis Hamman, American physician, 1877–1946. Mediastinal emphysema. *J. A. M. A.*, 1945, **128**: 1–6.

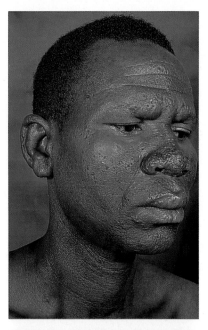

121 Lepromatous leprosy. This Nigerian farmer came with his brother because of concern over his changed appearance. There is diffuse infiltration and induration of the skin of the face especially the nose, lips and brows, where the eyebrows have been lost and fold formation is beginning to produce the classic leonine appearance. The ear has a swollen nodular appearance. The nasal mucosa is infiltrated and sneezing will produce an aerosol of lepra bacilli.

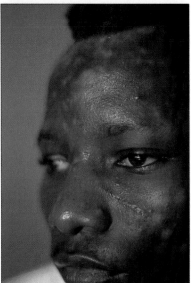

122 Leprosy (hypopigmented macules). The early lesions of borderline tuberculoid leprosy are macules with loss of pigment, which may be hypoaesthetic. A complete loss of pigment is not leprosy, but vitiligo. There was an associated thickened greater auricular nerve (*see* **547**).

FAT FACE—DRY AND MENTALLY SLOW

Myxoedema

The appearance of the face in hypothyroidism reflects many changes and is often recognised as the patient walks into the room. The apathy, pallor, thickened skin, puffy hands and face, thin hair, hoarse voice and slow actions may suggest the diagnosis. Vague symptoms of tiredness, aches and poor concentration should be mental prompts for considering the diagnosis. The 'before and after' pictures in this section demonstrate the classic appearance, which is best noted with hindsight!

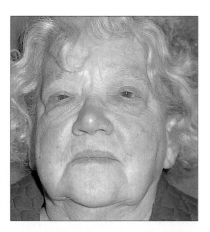

123 Myxoedema (fat face). The face is podgy and fat, and the eyebrows are thin. There is little else to note. Suspicion was confirmed by the slow tendon reflexes. This round stolid impassive appearance is as much sensed as seen and should raise the possibility of the diagnosis, especially when associated with vague, but important symptoms such as rheumatic pain, tiredness, lethargy and constipation.

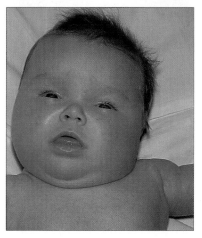

124 A hypothyroid infant. The child is inactive, sluggish, pasty-faced and constipated. The face is coarse, hair sparse, and skin cool. Prolonged physiological jaundice, constipation and feeding difficulties are the early signs in an infant. The classic facies of hypothyroidism can be seen across the ages of man (see **126, 127, 129, 131**). and the dissimilar similarity of trisomy 21 is shown in **125**. An apparent increase in tongue size (macroglossia) is seen in both the cretin and in Down's syndrome (trisomy 21).

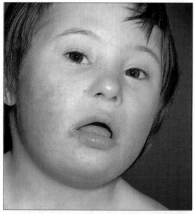

125 Down's syndrome.[17] Trisomy 21 is characterized by a round face, a big tongue, which may show fissures (*see* **341**), prominent epicanthic folds, a downward slope of the eyes to the midline, and a low nasal bridge. The hands are squat with a single transverse crease and may show incurving of the fifth finger.

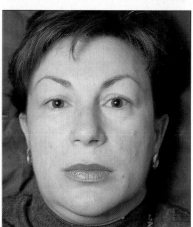

126a Myxoedema masquerading as hypercholesterolaemia. This short-sighted woman came from Portugal with a sheaf of lipid analyses and a complaint of nocturnal tingling of the hands. She took off her glasses, and her facies, which was puffy and pale, was confirmed as that of hypothyroidism by the sustained slow tendon reflexes. Her cholesterol fell from 700mgm% (18mmol/l) to 300mgm% (7.7 mmol/l) over four months on thyroxine.

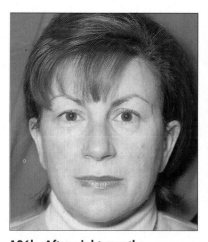

126b After eight months treatment. Her face has regained its natural contours, she is mentally alert (even her husband complains!) and aside from the obvious changes she says that for the first time in five years she has had to shave her legs—she had ascribed the hair loss to middle age.

[17]John Langdon Haydon Down, English physician at The Royal London Hospital, 1828–1891; described 1866.

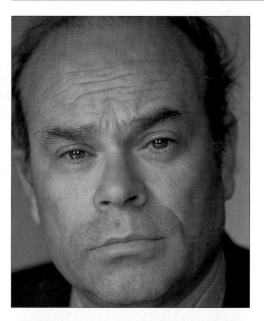

127 Hypothyroid male (facies). A man lost his drive, then found he was unable to concentrate and developed business difficulties. He went for medical screening and began treatment for 'depression' and a high serum cholesterol. It was nearly 18 months before his appearance and the secondary lipid changes were appreciated. A dull intellect and an insidious change in appearance with dry hair and puffy features could be normal.

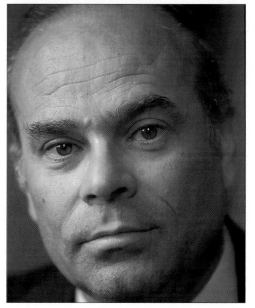

128 Hypothyroid man in 127 after treatment. Four months after starting thyroxine replacement therapy, this man was back to normal.

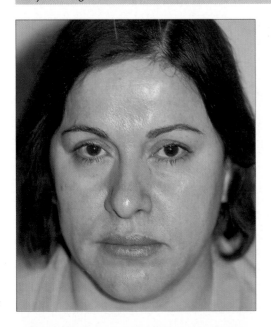

129 Hypothyroid female. This woman slept a great deal and complained of constipation.

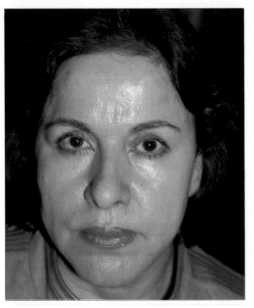

130 Hypothyroid woman in 129 after treatment. She no longer needed so much sleep after treatment!

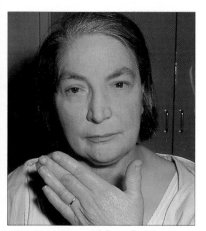

131 Hypothyroid female. This woman presented at a surgical clinic for varicose veins. The surgeon recognised the facies as she walked into the room and escorted her to his medical colleague!

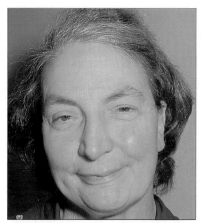

132 Hypothyroid female in 131 after treatment. The dull stolid look, dry hair and facial broadening was transformed after thyroid hormone therapy. The most striking features are the changed mental outlook and facial shape.

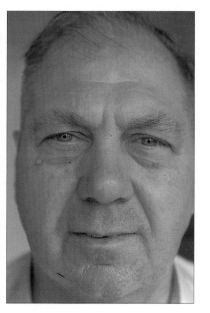

133 Hypothyroid male (sparse eyebrows). A man with depression, sparse eyebrows and a rounding of the face. Hair loss is a feature of myxoedema and may be reflected in thinning of the eyebrows or a curious mown-stubble appearance over the arms, hands or legs (*see* **419, 420**).

FAT AND PLETHORIC FACE

Many classic disease changes are insidious and may be dated by asking to see photographs in the patient's bag, wallet or photograph album. Photographs are an often untapped source of information.

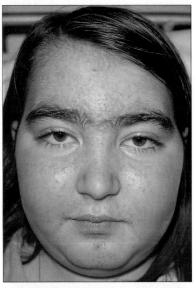

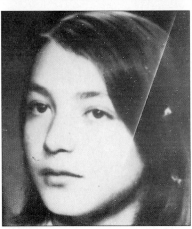

134 Cushing's syndrome[18] facies.
A teenage girl with an adrenal carcinoma. She has acne and hirsutes, greasy hair and skin, facial fat leading to the moon face and plethora due to the thin skin. The clinical picture occurs after long exposure to inappropriately elevated plasma glucocorticoid levels. The term *disease* refers to excessive corticotrophin secretion by a pituitary adenoma, while the *syndrome* is usually due to ectopic corticotrophin secretion by small cell lung cancers or indolent tumours elsewhere. The corticotrophin independent syndrome is produced by benign or malign adrenal tumours producing glucocorticoids. Excessive facial hair in malignant adrenal tumours reflects relative inefficiency of adrenal carcinomas at the synthesis of cortisol and overproduction of androgenic precursors. Adrenal adenomas tend to synthesise cortisol efficiently, which is clinically manifested as cortisol excess with weight gain, facial fat and marked supraclavicular fat pads, mild hirsutes, diabetes mellitus, hypertension, muscle weakness, acne, thin skin and thin bones.[19]

135. Passport photo of girl in 134 taken nine months earlier.

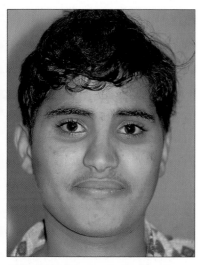

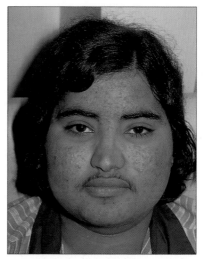

136 Early iatrogenic Cushing's syndrome. The effect of treatment with substantial corticosteroids over an eight-month period is seen in **137** and **138**.

137 Iatrogenic Cushing's syndrome (later).

138 Iatrogenic Cushing's syndrome (later still). The clinical features are now gross.

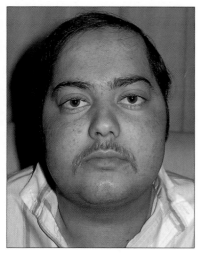

---

[18]The definitive paper written in 1932 by Harvey W. Cushing.
[19]Review of Cushing's syndrome. *N. Eng. J. Med.*, March 23 1995.

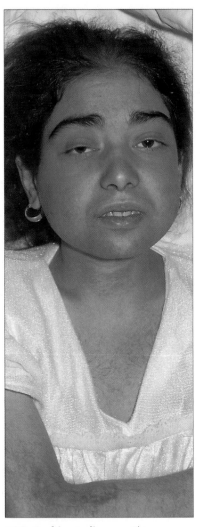

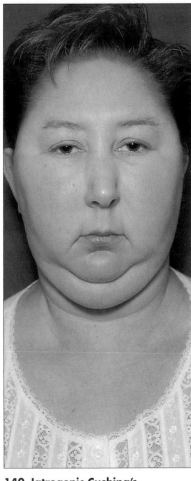

140 Iatrogenic Cushing's syndrome. This was secondary to treatment with prednisolone. Supraclavicular fat pads are a prominent feature.

139 Cushing's disease. This woman had muscle weakness with difficulty in rising when on the ground, mild facial hirsutes, livid striae (*see* **606**) on the arm and spontaneous bruising, as well as vertebral collapse due to osteoporosis.

THIN FACE

Loss of fat, muscle, and fluid may contribute to the appearance of thinness. A body mass index of less than 19–20 kg/Ht.m^2 may reflect female fashion, but as it falls further is unphysiological. Weight loss reflects an imbalance between intake and expenditure. Disease may lead to a loss of appetite and a fall in intake while catabolism continues. Infection and malignant disease with anorectic inflammatory mediators therefore lead to weight loss as may deliberate food restriction by the patient with anorexia nervosa.

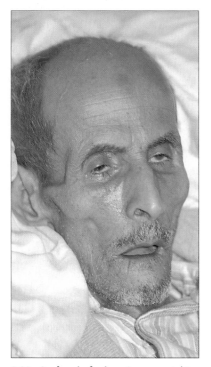

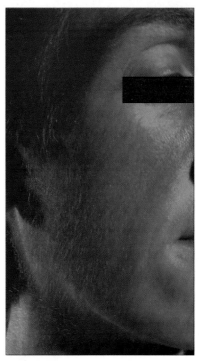

141 Cachexic facies. Severe weight loss in a patient with terminal disseminated gastric cancer. Anorexia aggravates the situation. Weakness and lethargy accounts for the fading prayer callus on the forehead because he is too weak to get out of bed and kneel to pray.

142 Facial hair in anorexia nervosa. Anorexia nervosa with severely limited energy intake. There is a typical increase in fine lanugo hair on the cheeks and a dry cold skin.

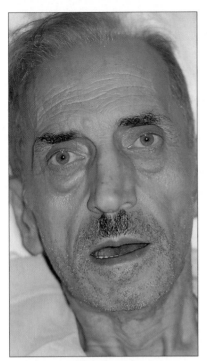

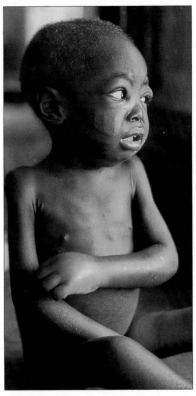

143 Thin, ill and jaundiced. An appreciation of illness and health comes from observing the component parts. Jaundice seen in the conjunctivae, dehydration and severe weight loss are all features here in this patient with carcinoma of the pancreas.

144 Kwashiorkor[20] face and habitus. Kwashiorkor is an acute illness occurring in individuals with inadequate nutrition and often with a preceding acute infection. Apathy, misery, oedema, and skin changes are the striking characteristic clinical features. There is periorbital oedema and abdominal swelling.

---

[20]Ghanaian word for the changeling or displaced child—the illness that the deposed baby gets when the next child is born and takes the breast milk. The changeling then loses his source of protein and lives on carbohydrate and at ground level because he is no longer slung on his mother's back. As a result he is prone to infection.

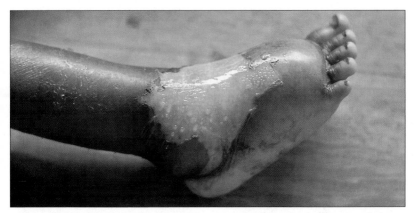

145 Kwashiorkor leg and skin (eczema craquelé). The skin becomes darker, dry and thin, and cracks like the craquelure of an old painting (or crazy paving) and peels away, leaving a hypopigmented patch. This may be seen in adult malnutrition from any cause.

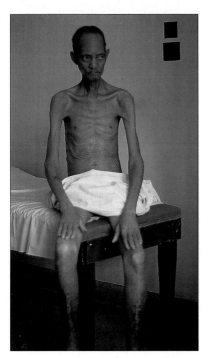

146 Adult malnutrition. The changes on the skin of the legs mirror the skin changes in kwashiorkor.

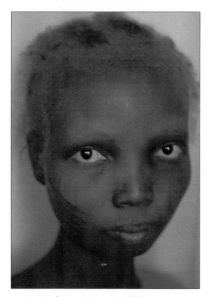

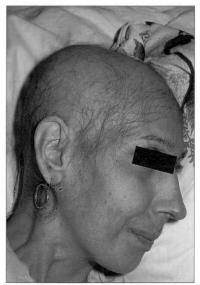

147 Malnutrition adult face and hair. The hair becomes thin, and loses its curl and colour.

148 Hair loss in illness. This patient has severe ulcerative colitis. Any severe illness may be associated with telogen effluvium.

149 Dystrophia myotonica. The face may be thin because the facial, masseter, temporalis and sternomastoid muscles are wasted. Bilateral ptosis may be a feature and frontal balding may be seen in men.

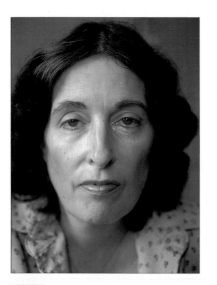

SWEATY AND IRRITABLE

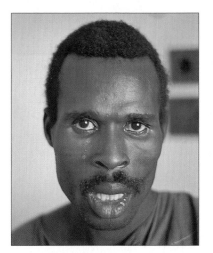

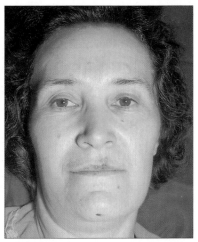

150 The febrile patient. This Nigerian man is ill with lobar pneumonia and a temperature of 40°C. He is hot, sweaty, his eyes are slightly sunken and his face is apathetic; he has a tinge of jaundice. Abnormal liver function is common in pneumococcal infection, and even more common in *Legionella* infections.

151 Herpes labialis in pneumococcal pneumonia. This woman is recovering from pneumonia. Herpes simplex infection on the lip may be seen in as many as 30% of patients. It frequently accompanies fever.

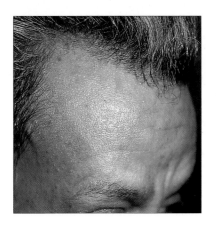

152 Hypoglycaemia and sweating in November (U.K.). If a patient becomes angry at being kept waiting and then aggressive at lunch time in a medical outpatients unit this may be reasonable and need addressing, but copious sweating in midwinter may have a medical cause! The pallor and cold, wet, feel to the hand with a fast pulse is typical. This insulin-dependent diabetic needed his lunch!

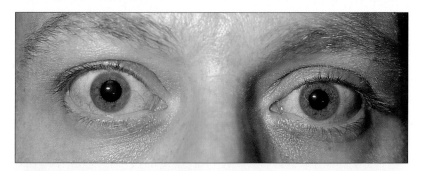

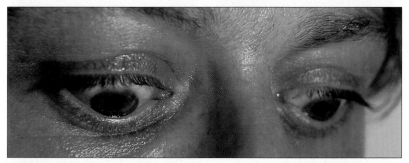

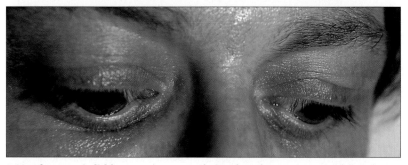

153 Thyrotoxic lid lag. 'Look up at my fingers for a few moments and follow them as they move downwards.' The patient shown here and the patient in **154** show the phenomenon of lid lag—there is a moment before the upper lid catches up with the globe. In both series there is lid lag, but the myotonic individual in **154** shows no other signs to suggest thyrotoxicosis. 'Could there be another cause because I can see nothing except lid lag?' In contrast the man in **153** has a sweaty skin, periorbital puffiness and some conjunctival injection, all of which back up a diagnosis of thyrotoxicosis. Only one sign means you should look for confirmatory evidence to back up your first thought.

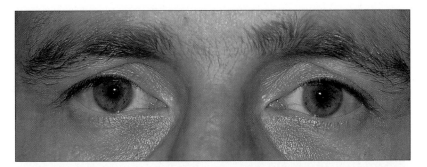

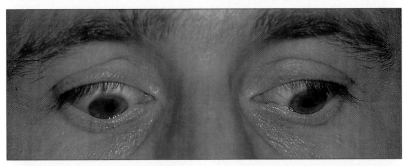

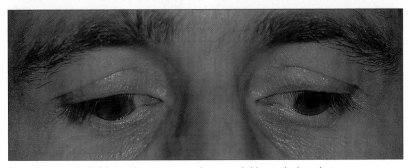

154 Myotonic lid lag. This patient's only sign is lid lag, which is due to myotonia—the muscle once stimulated remains contracted. The delay in letting go may be noticed when shaking hands and may be worse with cold and after exertion. This man's children could not swim in the sea in winter because they became stiff.

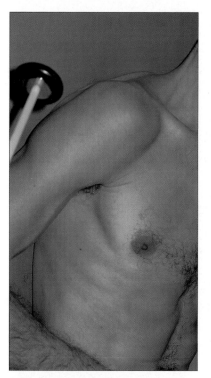

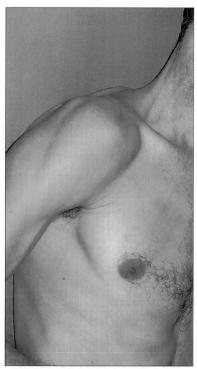

155 Myotonia before a tap with a patellar hammer. Myotonia describes the continued contraction of a muscle after the effort or stimulus has ceased. It is due to an abnormality of the muscle fibre and is seen in myotonia congenita (Thomsen's[21] disease) without muscle wasting or indeed without hypertrophy; in dystrophia myotonica with wasting; and prominently in paramyotonia after exposure to cold. A variant of myotonia congenita may be associated with malignant hyperthermia.

156 Myotonia after a tap with a patellar hammer. All forms of myotonia are inherited in an autosomal dominant manner. It may also be drug-induced and appear as a symptom complicating motor neurone disease and polymyositis.

---

[21]Asmus Julius Thomas Thomsen, Danish physician, 1815–1896; described it in himself and his family. Thomsen J. Tonische Krämpfe in willkürlich bewegliche Muskein in Folge von ererbter psychischer Disposition (ataxia muscularis?). *Arch. Psychiat.* (Berlin), 1875–76, **6**. pp.706–718.

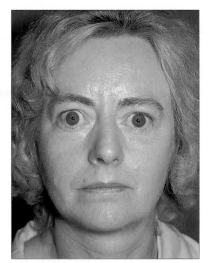

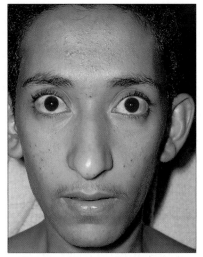

157 Thyrotoxicosis (Caucasian face). As a result of thyrotoxicosis this lady is overwrought and has heat intolerance. She is tense and sweaty, and her eyes show lid retraction and proptosis. The ocular features affect the right eye more than the left, and the sclera is visible above the right iris.

158 Thyrotoxicosis (Arab face). This youth shows bilateral symmetrical lid retraction and the sclerae are visible above and below the iris. In normal people the sclerae may be exposed below the iris if the gaze is fixed above the horizontal plane.

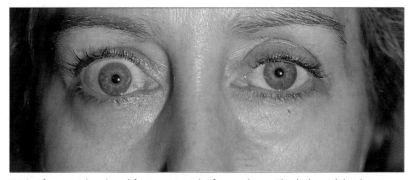

159 Thyrotoxicosis with asymmetrical eye signs. This lady said that her husband had noticed her left ptosis! In fact her right eye is proptosed and the lid retracted so that the sclera is visible above the iris. On the left the sclera is just seen below the iris and this has little significance diagnostically. Conjunctival vessels are present, and her skin glistens because she feels the heat.

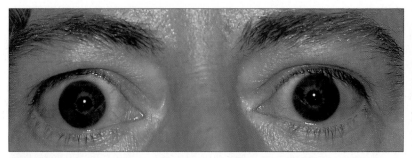

160 Ill thyrotoxic woman. This woman's thyrotoxicosis had led to weight loss, tension, lid retraction (greater on the left) and a sweaty skin.

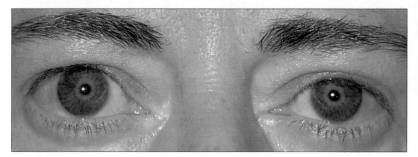

161 Thyrotoxic woman after carbimazole. The woman in **160** is now euthyroid after two weeks' treatment with carbimazole. Her lid retraction and tension have diminished.

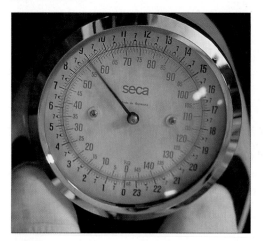

162 The scales sign. A man complained of anxiety and insomnia. His minor eye signs were masked by glasses and the significance of his fidgeting was missed. However, when he stood on the scales the tip of the pointer trembled and would not settle. Fine oscillation continued and the relevance of his history was finally understood! He was thyrotoxic, the oscillations reflecting his cardiac high output state. The weighing scales were acting as a crude ballistocardiograph!

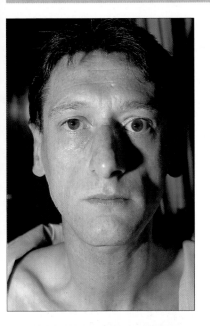

163 Ill thyrotoxic man. This man had palpitations and weight loss despite eating. He is thin and sweaty. On the left side there is proptosis and lid retraction.

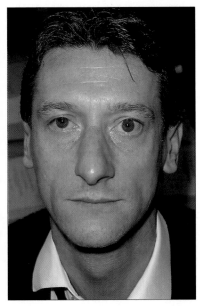

164 Thyrotoxic man after thyroidectomy. The man in **163** is now euthyroid and he has regained his lost weight. The eye signs and tensions are less marked.

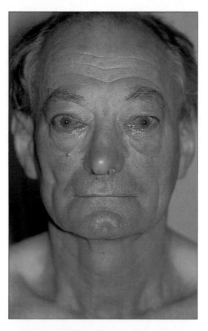

165 Severe ophthalmopathy in thyrotoxicosis. This chauffeur uncharacteristically lost his temper in a traffic jam and so his employer sent him to his doctor. He has the eye signs of Graves'[22] disease—periorbital oedema, chemosis, conjunctival injection and lid retraction. Proptosis is more marked for the right eye and he has difficulty closing his right eyelid and therefore a potential for right corneal damage (*see* **166**). The proptosis is disguised by chemosis and the vascular injection of the sclera, particularly laterally near the lateral rectus insertion.

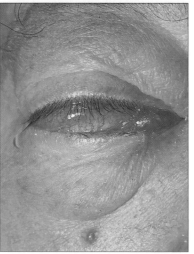

166 The proptosed eye does not close. The man in **165** is unable to close his right eye. There is therefore a danger of corneal damage because blinking is impaired and the cornea may become dry.

[22]Robert James Graves, Irish physician, 1795–1853. New observed affection of the thyroid gland in females. *Lond. Med. Surg. J.*, 1835, 516–17.

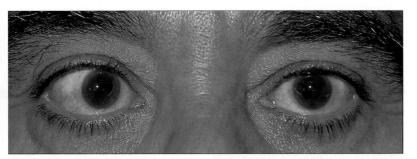

167 Eyes with ocular muscle involvement in ophthalmic Graves' disease.
This man was initially euthyroid, but has a slight right-sided proptosis. He had thyroid
autoantibodies and a raised thyroid stimulating hormone level. Over 12 months he
became hypothyroid and developed progressive ophthalmoplegia.

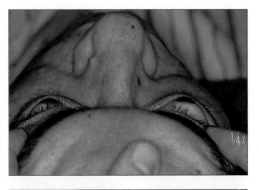

**168 Eyes with uni-
lateral proptosis and
computerised tomo-
graphic scan of the
orbits.** The slight proptosis of
the right eye is best seen from
above and the swollen eye
muscles can be appreciated on
the scan. Swelling of the
orbital contents may lead to
optic nerve compression,
especially if decompressive
protrusion does not occur.

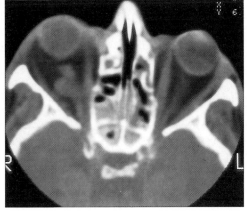

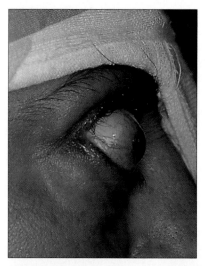

169 Malignant exophthalmos: lateral view. Protrusion of the eye leads to failure of the upper lid to sweep the cornea on blinking, leading to dryness and a risk of corneal damage. A lateral tarsorrhaphy has been performed to protect the left cornea. Progressive swelling of the orbital contents may lead to optic nerve damage and visual loss.

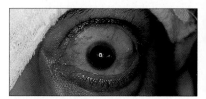

170 Malignant exophthalmos: front view.

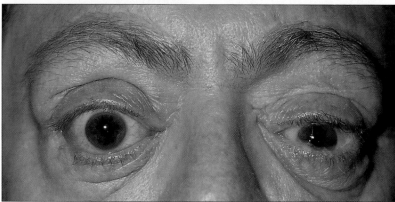

171 Treated malignant exophthalmos. A dusty holiday in Egypt touring archaeological sites was cut short by a painful sore left eye. This man wore dark glasses and removed them to display these signs—seen here after examination. He has periorbital oedema, conjunctival injection, right-sided eye lid retraction and proptosis, inferior displacement of the left globe, and a discharge. Is this the gross picture of acute or acute-on-chronic ophthalmic Graves' disease? If the lateral aspects of the eye fissures are examined, it can be seen that bilateral tarrsorrhaphies have been performed long ago—so the problem is long-standing. In addition, scars in the eyebrows reflect orbital decompression operations. So this is chronic treated malignant eye disease, and the defective wiper effect in dusty conditions led to corneal abrasion. The 'discharge' is fluoroscein stain used to check for epithelial damage.

ASYMMETRY OF MOVEMENT

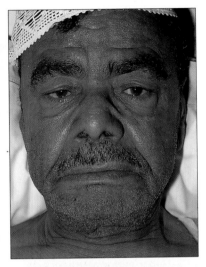

172 Upper motor neurone facial palsy at rest. The weakness is predominantly of the lower face because the forehead is bilaterally innervated. The lesion lies above the facial nucleus. A stroke left this man with a mild right-sided hemiplegia. All that is seen is a slight droop at the right corner of the mouth. He has a corneal arcus.

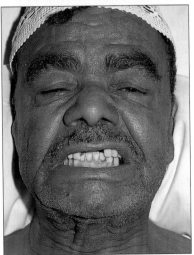

173 Upper motor neurone facial palsy—'Show your teeth'[23] When asked to show his teeth both sides of this man's mouth move, but the right side is less mobile.

---

[23]Teeth come either from God, the Government or the market place, so patients may take them out and show you. As you ask them to show you their teeth make the movement you want them to make!

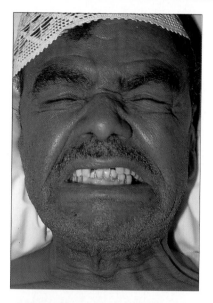

174 Upper motor neurone facial palsy—'Show your teeth'—'Try harder'—to show unilateral platysma action. When asked to try harder and to screw up his eyes at the same time this man has no upper facial weakness, minimal weakness of the right lower face and weakness of the right platysma. The platysma is in action on the left side, but not on the right.

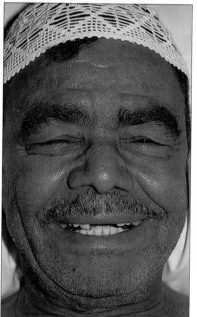

175 Upper motor neurone facial palsy—the effect of emotion and smiling. All the attention and being asked to whistle makes this man smile and the emotional act produces a much more normal movement of the mouth. The movement of the involved side may be exaggerated and this is a specific feature of an upper motor neurone lesion. In this situation any hemiplegia will be on the same side and a hemianopia will indicate a hemisphere lesion.

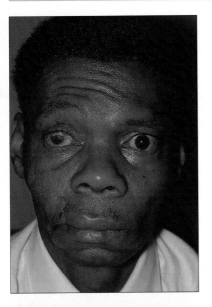

176 Lower motor neurone facial palsy at rest. There is flaccid weakness of all the muscles on the left side of the face. The upper face is weak and there is a failure of forehead wrinkles to appear on raising the eyebrows. The palpebral fissure is widened, yet the eyebrow droops, and there is loss of the nasolabial fold. Both the upper and lower face are affected and the weakness includes both voluntary and emotional movement.

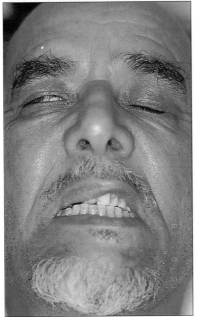

177 Lower motor neurone facial palsy—'Show your teeth and close your eyes'. The eyelid remains open and the eye ball rolls up and out. This is Bell's[24] phenomenon.

[24]Sir Charles Bell, 1774–1842. On the nerves; giving an account of some experiments on their structure and functions, which lead to a new arrangement of the system. *Philos. Tr. Roy. Soc.* (London), 1821, **111**; 398–424.

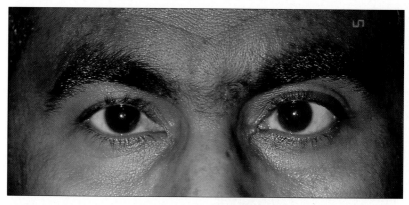

178 Lower motor neurone facial palsy—Bell's palsy. Mild palsies may be missed. The weak left face is not obvious, but the palpebral fissure is widened.

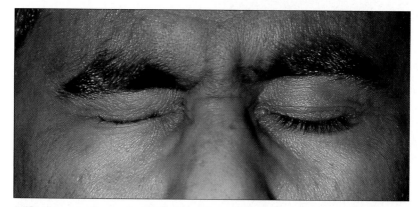

179 Lower motor neurone facial palsy—'Screw up your eyes'. This reveals the mild Bell's palsy. Note the difference in length of the visible eye-lashes on the affected side. Be aware of the loss of spontaneous blinking on that side. The site of the lesion may lie anywhere from the nucleus in the pons onwards: if it is associated with a sixth nerve palsy it is pontine; if with fifth and eighth nerve palsies the lesion is in the cerebellopontine angle; if sound is distorted by the loss of automatic gain reduction from paralysis of the stapedius muscle attenuating intense noise-and taste is affected, the lesion lies between the brain stem and chorda tympani. Check for herpetic vesicles in the ear (*see* **277**)—herpes zoster involving the geniculate ganglion produces the Ramsay Hunt syndrome.[25]

---

[25]Ramsay Hunt J. On herpetic inflammation of the geniculate ganglion. A new syndrome and its complications. *J. Nerv. Ment. Dis.*, 1907, **34**: 73–6.

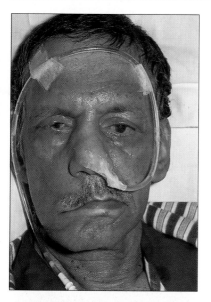

180 Lower motor neurone facial palsy and deafness. This man with a cerebellopontine-angle acoustic neuroma has a lower motor neurone facial palsy (due to seventh cranial nerve involvement), corneal anaesthesia needing a tarsorrhaphy to protect it (due to fifth cranial nerve involvement), and is deaf in the right ear (due to eighth cranial nerve involvement).

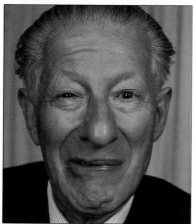

181 Bilateral lower motor neurone facial palsy—'Close your eyes and show your teeth'. This may be overlooked because of the symmetry, even on attempted movement. But emotional paralysis leads to a mask-like face (*see* **189**), which is transformed by smiling.

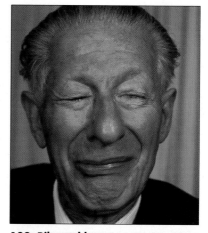

182 Bilateral lower motor neurone facial palsy—'Please try harder!' The smile is still very weak. Compare the eyelashes here and in **179**. Bilateral palsy may occur in infective polyneuritis, progressive muscular atrophy and sarcoid-osis. Myasthenia should be excluded.

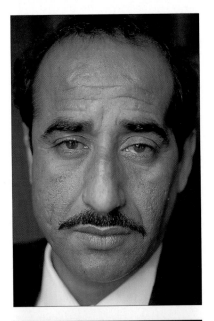

183 Trigeminal (fifth cranial) nerve motor palsy with wasting of masseter and temporalis. This man has a trigeminal nerve neuroma with a complete trigeminal nerve palsy. He has temporal fossa and cheek wasting caused by a lower motor neurone lesion affecting the temporalis, masseter and pterygoid muscles (*see* **184**). Note the slight conjunctival injection on the left where the corneal reflex is absent.

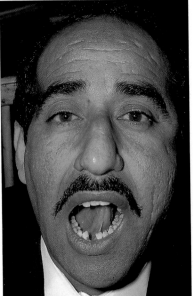

184 Trigeminal (fifth cranial) nerve motor palsy—'Open your mouth!' The jaw deviates away from the weak side on opening the mouth because the pterygoids on the unaffected side are unopposed.

WEAKNESS, HYPERTONICITY AND SPASM

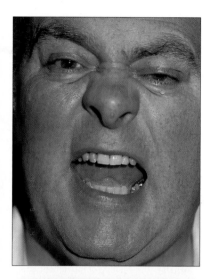

185 Facial fatigue. This man—a lover of steak—said he had to help his lower jaw chew through meat with the aid of his hand. He has been fixing his gaze at the ceiling for as long as he could; as he fatigued bilateral ptosis developed. The effort to smile shows the 'myasthenic snarl'.

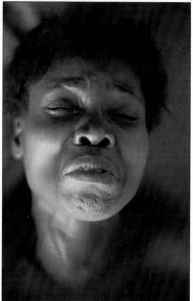

186 Risus sardonicus. Late at night in a Nigerian hospital casualty department a door slammed and this woman stiffened (*see* **516**). The alae nasi, the muscles at the angles of the mouth and those that lift the eye brows, as well as the platysma and sternomastoids are all contracted in a fixed humourless grimace. This is a severe tetanic spasm. A fixed risus may also occur in strychnine poisoning, as a hysterical manifestation, and in malingerers.

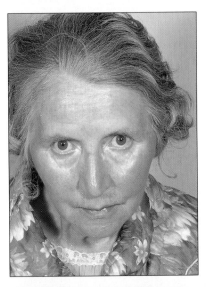

187 The immobile face. The face devoid of expression belies the activity within. The neck is flexed and tense sternomastoids stand out. The face is sweaty and greasy, yet blinking is minimal and there seems to be a surprised look. Bilateral emotional palsy often transformed with a smile is typically seen in Parkinson's[26] disease (paralysis agitans) and pseudobulbar palsy.

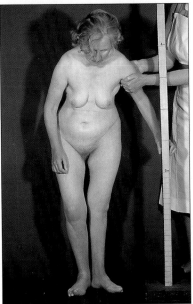

188 Parkinson's disease (body habitus). The paucity of movement and its restricted sweep show itself in the shuffling gait—the head is bent forward, the posture is stooped and rigid, the arm is adducted and fails to swing spontaneously with the gait. As she enters, the speed of her walk increases until she seems to run, due to her festinant gait (*festinare* L. To hasten), and as she turns to sit the movement is made with the body as one piece.

[26]Sir James Parkinson, 1755–1824. An essay on the shaking palsy., Whittingham and Rowland, London, 1817.

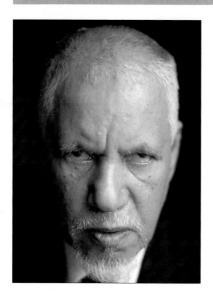

189 Parkinson's disease (a male face and an 'invisible pillow'). The cardinal features of Parkinson's disease are tremor, rigidity and akinesia. Facial muscle immobility leads to a fixed flat expression devoid of emotion. This man dribbled excessively and found swallowing required effort. His head is bent forwards as if by a pillow so that to gaze at the camera he has to look upwards. This is unlike an oculogyric crisis in which the gaze is fixed upward and which may occur in postencephalitic Parkinson's disease, phenothiazine toxicity, hysteria and hypoparathyroidism.

COMPONENTS OF THE FACE

The eyes

The eyes include the surrounding skin and eyebrows, the lids and orbit, and the eye itself— the conjunctiva, sclera, cornea, iris, pupil and fundus.

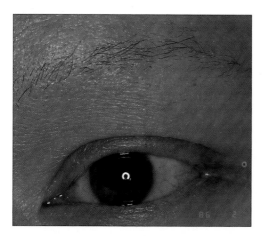

190 Alopecia areata affecting the eyebrow and eyelashes. Broken 'exclamation mark' hairs can be seen in the eyebrow and eyelashes. The scalp (*see* **98**) is the usual site, but men may complain of patches in the beard or eyebrow. Loss of eyebrows may be due to an endocrine disorder (e.g. hypothyroidism, *see* **133**), infection (e.g. lepromatous leprosy, *see* **121**), cosmetic plucking (*see* **237**), or related to disease of the hair follicle.

PTOSIS[27]

Ptosis may result from muscle, motor nerve end plate or cranial and sympathetic nerve disease, involving the smooth or striated muscle fibres of levator palpebrae superioris. It may affect one or both sides. If unilateral, is it partial ptosis seen **relative** to the unaffected side?—if so a Horner's syndrome[28] is the first diagnostic choice. If the ptosis is **absolutely** obvious and there is no need to refer to the other eye, the first diagnostic choice is a third cranial nerve palsy. Decide after examining the pupil size and looking for the presence of a squint. Other causes may be unilateral or bilateral and will be differentiated by the clinical context. Tabetic ptosis is bilateral. A provisional diagnosis may be attempted from across the room.

Is the ptosis:
- Unilateral or bilateral?
- Relative or absolute?[29]

Unilateral ptosis may be congenital or due to myasthenia or trauma and surgery. Alternatively the ptosis may be a 'pseudoptosis' (*see* **207**).

Bilateral ptosis may be congenital or due to myasthenia, myopathy, dystrophia myotonica, tabes dorsalis or a bilateral Horner's syndrome.

If there is frontalis muscle overaction, look to see on which side. If the ptosis is functional, it will be on the opposite side to the ptosis.

---

[27]Greek. Adverb: falling or prolapsus.

[28]Johann Friedrich Horner, 1831–1886. Uber eine form von Ptosis. *Klin. Mbl. Augen-heilk*, 1869, **7**:193–8. Claude Bernard described this syndrome in 1862.

[29]These terminologies *may* help in analysis. **Relative** implies that you decide by comparing with the other side and **absolute** is obvious even if only one eye is seen. The ptosis of Horner's syndrome is relative and that of third nerve palsy is usually absolute. ***Partial or complete*** are alternative terms, but if one thinks that it is complete and that the eye is shut, this may not be so. Look for the iris limbus: it may just be seen (*see* **211**) and confirm deviation down and outwards—you have to look carefully. Some causes are less likely to be absolute/complete than relative/partial. An absolute ptosis may be congenital, myopathic or myasthenic; if unilateral it is more likely to be due to a third nerve palsy, but could be due to one of the former causes. A relative unilateral ptosis is usually due to a Horner's syndrome. Bilateral partial ptosis may also be tabetic, but it could—just—be a bilateral Horner's syndrome!

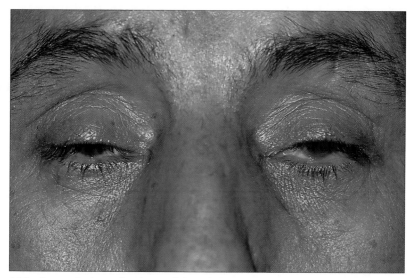

191 Congenital ptosis. This is a bilateral obvious ptosis. but it may be unilateral.

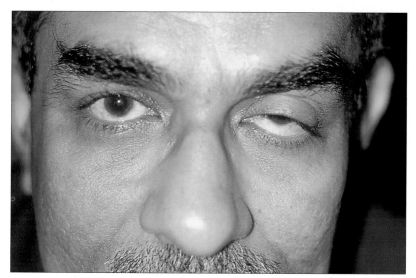

192 Unilateral congenital ptosis. A third nerve palsy can be excluded because the eye is not deviated.

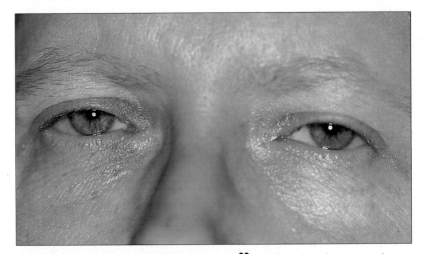

193 Tabes dorsalis and Argyll Robertson[30] pupils. Bilateral ptosis may be accompanied by overaction of the frontalis to give a surprised appearance. The pupils are small and irregular (*see* **245**).

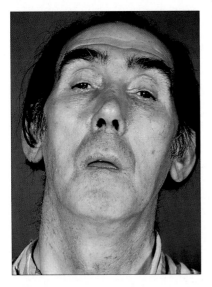

194 Dystrophia myotonica and bilateral ptosis. This man has frontal balding, a myopathic facies with wasted facial muscles, and a sagging mouth. He has extended his neck so that he can see from beneath his lowered lids. His neck muscles are thin. Myotonia (*see* **155**) was present.

[30]Douglas Moray Cooper Lamb Argyll Robertson, 1837–1909. Robertson, A. On an interesting series of eye symptoms in a case of spinal disease, with remarks on the action of belladonna on the iris. *Edin. Med. J.*, 1868, **14**: 696–708.

MYASTHENIA GRAVIS.

Myasthenia gravis is characterised by a varying unilateral or bilateral ptosis, which is seen alone or with weakness of other cranial nerves.

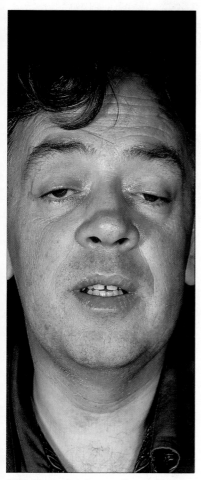

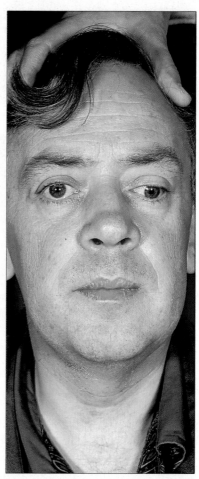

195 Myasthenia gravis and bilateral ptosis. Slight frontalis overaction and weakness of the mouth were accompanied by diplopia after prolonged upward gaze.

196 Myaesthenia gravis and bilateral ptosis after edrophonium injection. The ptosis improved, though the third cranial nerve weakness remains (i.e. the eye squints down and outwards).

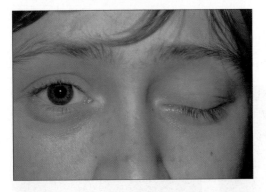

197 Myasthenia gravis and unilateral ptosis. Logic does not apply—unilateral ptosis frequently accompanies myasthenia. Before injection of edrophonium there is an absolute, but not totally complete, ptosis. The iris is seen in the fissure, the limbus is deviated laterally, and the corneal protrusion is depressed.

198 Myasthenia gravis after edrophonium chloride injection. A residual third nerve weakness is seen.

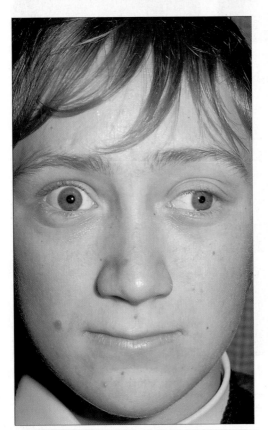

THE EFFECT OF FATIGUE IN MYASTHENIA GRAVIS IS CHARACTERISTIC.

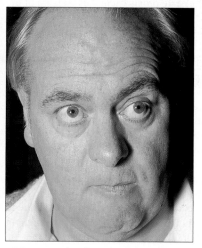

199 Myasthenia gravis 1—'Look up'.

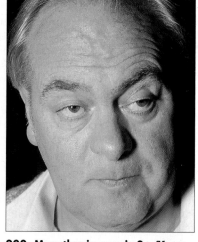

200 Myasthenia gravis 2—'Keep looking up'. The ptosis appears and the frontalis overaction diminishes.

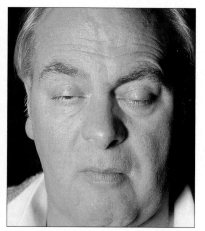

201 Myasthenia gravis 3—'Keep looking up'. The ptosis becomes even more marked and the frontalis furrowing diminishes as fatigue increases. The upward gaze cannot be maintained.

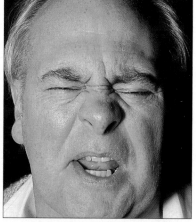

202 Myasthenia gravis 4—'Now... show your teeth and screw up your eyes'. Finally the weakness produces the characteristic snarl and inability to bury the eyelashes.

HORNER'S SYNDROME

Horner's syndrome is characterised by a relative ptosis caused by a lesion of the sympathetic supply to the eye. It consists of:

- Partial ptosis due to paralysis of the smooth muscle of levator palpebrae superioris.
- Enophthalmos (always mentioned and difficult to see).
- A small regular pupil due to loss of supply to the dilator of the pupil.
- Absent sweating of the face if the lesion is below the bifurcation of the carotid artery where the fibres concerned with sweating separate.

The sympathetic fibres run downwards from the nucleus through the brain stem to the spinal cord and exit at T1. They ascend with the carotid artery through the carotid canal and reach the eye via the long ciliary nerve. The lesion can therefore be within the brain (e.g. haemorrhage), within the spinal cord (e.g. tumour), or peripheral (e.g. tumours or trauma of the sympathetic chain as it passes upwards with the carotid artery through the carotid canal and into the siphon to join the nerve to dilator pupillae). **203–209** show examples of Horner's syndrome due to four different causes, all of which are deducible from the setting or the signs— but you only see what you have taught yourself to see!

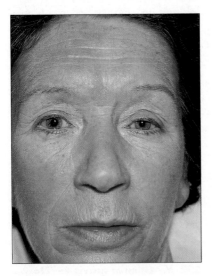

203 Horner's syndrome and pain down the left arm. This lady was a heavy cigarette smoker. She had wasting of the small muscles of the hand, a left ptosis and a small pupil. Chest radiography revealed a left apical carcinoma—a Pancoast[31] superior sulcus tumour.

---

[31]Henry Khunrath Pancoast, radiologist, 1875–1939. Superior pulmonary sulcus tumour. *J. A. M. A.*, 1932, **99**: 1391–96. But antedated by his clinical colleague W. Freeman. Endothelioma of pleura simulating spinal cord tumour. *Int. Clin. Ser.*, 1921, **31(4)**:159–66. Pancoast was the radiologist in the first case, but missed the diagnosis.

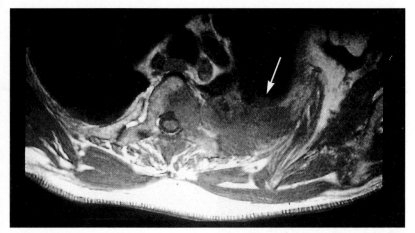

204 Magnetic resonance image showing a Pancoast tumour of the lung.
The lung tumour has invaded the rib and vertebral body, and involves the first thoracic root and sympathetic chain.

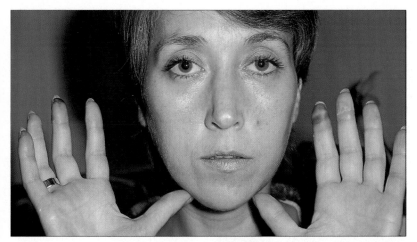

205 A hairdresser from Holloway with headaches. This lady had bilateral digital ischaemia, which was worse on the left, a left-sided ptosis and a small pupil. The lid met the pupil tangentially on both sides and she had left frontalis overaction. She might have migraine, which can lead to ptosis or have taken excess ergotamine and developed arterial spasm, while a cord lesion such as syringomyelia can lead to burns and ptosis. In fact she had severe Raynaud's disease leading to digital ischaemia. A sympathectomy was performed on the most affected side.

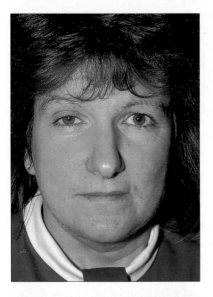

206 A nurse with relative ptosis and a small pupil. She has a thyroidectomy scar, which is just visible in the neck. Her Horner's syndrome is due to surgical damage to the sympathetic chain.

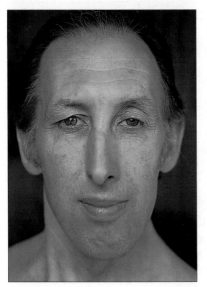

207 Right pseudoptosis[32] and apparent facial asymmetry. This man presented with hoarseness due to vagal palsy. A lax right upper lid simulates ptosis, but there is a left ptosis and the laxity is taken up by slight frontalis overaction. The pupil cannot be seen, but there is no other sign and it is likely that this is a Horner's syndrome. Facial asymmetry is due to the appearance of dramatic left sternomastoid wasting due to a lower motor neurone lesion of the spinal accessory nerve. The level can be deduced—at the base of the skull the spinal accessory nerve passes through the jugular foramen close to the hypoglossal foramen of the 12th cranial nerve and the carotid canal anteriorly. This man has jugular foramen syndrome. The hypoglossal nerve may also be involved—so look in the mouth (*see* **208**).

[32]Apparent or pseudoptosis may be due to laxity of the upper lid, or actual lid retraction on the other side may make the normal lid seem ptosed by comparison.

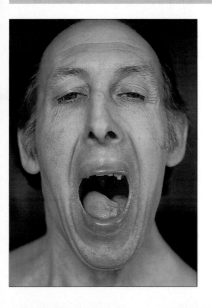

208 Horner's syndrome—'Open your mouth'. There is wasting of the left tongue due to a lower motor neurone 12th nerve lesion. The level must be at the base of the skull because the 12th nerve is involved.

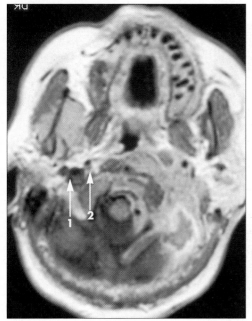

209 Magnetic resonance imaging scan of the base of the skull showing tumour at the jugular foramen. The head is not positioned straight because the teeth are cut obliquely. The tumour at the skull base surrounds the jugular foramen, which transmits the glossopharyngeal, vagus and spinal accessory nerves, and the hypoglossal foramen, and extends into the skull. All four lower cranial nerves are often involved together. (1=Carotid canal, 2=Jugular foramen)

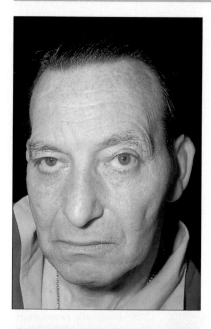

210 Functional ptosis. This man complains of a right-sided drooping of his eyelid. His pupils are normal and he has frontalis overaction on the opposite side to the ptosis, which raises the possibility that the ptosis may be functional since it is difficult to simulate a ptosis without some elevation of the opposite eyebrow. There may be spasm of orbicularis oculi on the affected side.

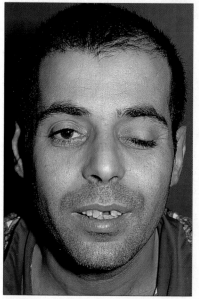

211 Unilateral ptosis. This is an obvious ptosis, so it may be congenital, myopathic, or due to a third nerve lesion. The ptosis is 'complete', but the eye is not totally shut—the sclera is seen between the palpebral fissure where the dark iris should be. The eye is deviated, so this ptosis is due to a third nerve lesion.

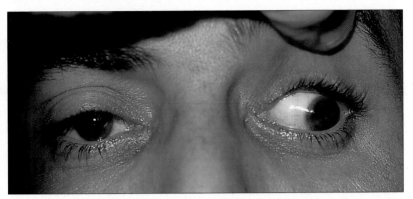

212 Third nerve palsy. This is confirmed on lifting the eyelid (palsy due to loss of the motor supply to levator palpebrae superioris) of the patient in **211**, when the down and outwards displacement is seen. The third cranial nerve has a long intracranial course—from the **n**ucleus passing through the **m**idbrain, then exits **i**nterpeduncularly and passes into the **c**avernous sinus and thence into the **o**rbit; **d**iabetes mellitus may be a cause of an isolated palsy. If the course is remembered—'**n**o **m**ore **i**gnorance **c**oming **o**ut, **d**octor!'—it is simpler to recall the possible pathologies that may occur in each section. The pupil is larger than its fellow and fixed to light due to loss of parasympathetic constrictor fibres and ennervations. The downward deviation is due to unopposed action of the superior oblique muscle, which is supplied by the fourth cranial nerve. The outwards deviation is due to the unopposed action of the lateral rectus (sixth cranial or abducens nerve).

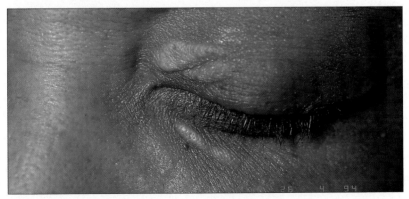

213 Eyelid with xanthelasma. The yellow plaque consists of lipid deposited in the skin. They may occur in familial hypercholesterolaemia at a young age, but are often absent. They may also be seen in polygenic hypercholesterolaemia, liver disease and hypothyroidism, as well as in individuals in middle age with a normal cholesterol. They are a sign of little value!

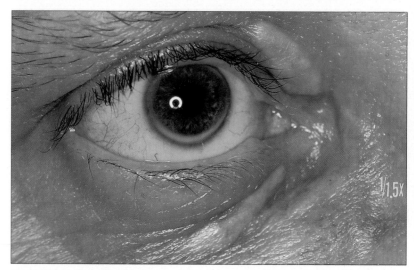

214 Xanthelasma and arcus. This patient's serum cholesterol is 5.4 mmol/l. A corneal arcus is a product of lipid deposition and may be partial or complete. It occurs more frequently in familial hypercholesterolaemia at a young age, but in middle age may have little significance. It is more valuable as a prompt to review the risk factors for coronary artery disease.

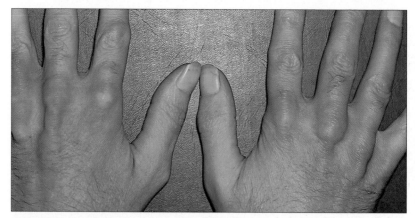

215 Tendon xanthomas. These feel bony because they are fibrotic. They are also seen at the patellar insertion on the tibial tubercle and in the Achilles tendon. They are the hallmark of familial hypercholesterolaemia, which is dominantly inherited and leads to a serum cholesterol of 9–11 mmol/l.. The frequency of heterozygotes in the United Kingdom is 1in 500. A corneal arcus is often absent.

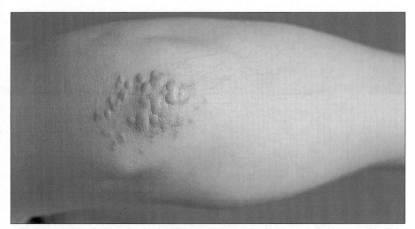

216 Eruptive xanthomas on the elbow (*see* 795a). Lipid deposition in the skin (xanthoma tuberosum) may be seen in youth in homozygous familial hyper-cholesterolaemia and affect the buttocks and palms. There is also joint involvement.

THE RED EYE
A red eye may have a local or a systemic cause.

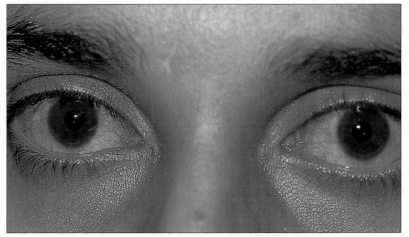

217 Acute conjunctivitis. There are many causes of conjunctivitis. The conjunctiva is inflamed and there is a pale ring at the corneal junction. There is no pain and no photophobia. Vision is not impaired.

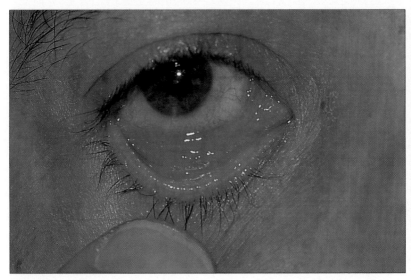

218 Chemosis. Inflammation may lead to oedema of the conjunctiva. This is often seen in thyroid eye disease.

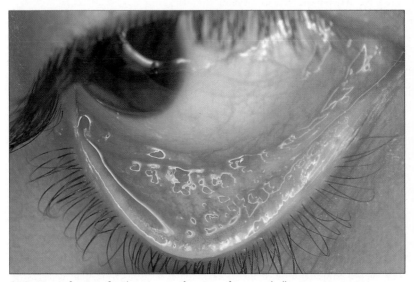

219 Vernal catarrh. This is a manifestation of seasonal allergic conjunctivitis.

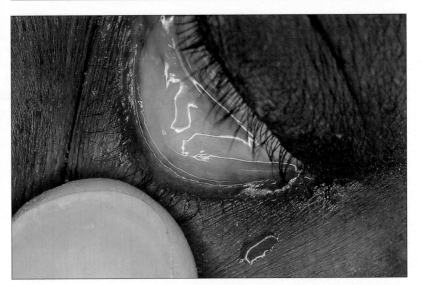

220 The conjunctiva as a gauge of anaemia. The conjunctiva in an anaemic Afro-Caribbean man. The capillary nailbed of the examiner is acting as a control.

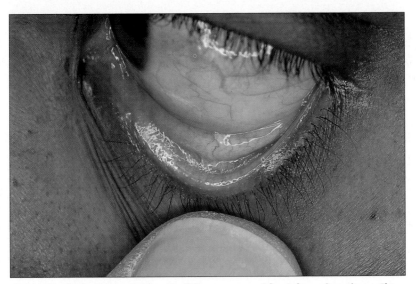

221 Less dark-skinned Afro-Caribbean man with pink conjunctivae. This man is not anaemic. The capillary nail bed of the examiner is acting as a control.

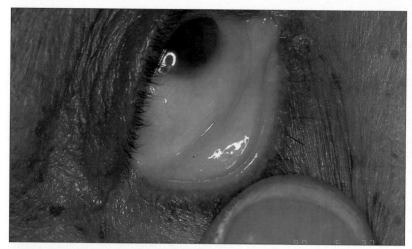

222 Pallor of the conjunctiva. This may give an indication of anaemia. This Indian woman has leukaemia. Compare with the control capillary nail bed.

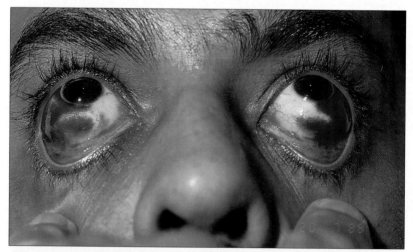

223 Bilateral subconjunctival haemorrhages. These may occur spontaneously in health for no apparent reason, but may follow prolonged coughing, vomiting or asphyxia. They are also associated with thrombolytic therapy and blood dyscrasias.

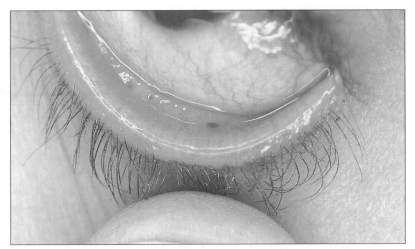

224 Conjunctival haemorrhage. A small embolus from bacterial endocarditis has lodged in the conjunctival vessels in the lower fornix. Abnormal bleeding is often seen in the unsupported conjunctival vessels.

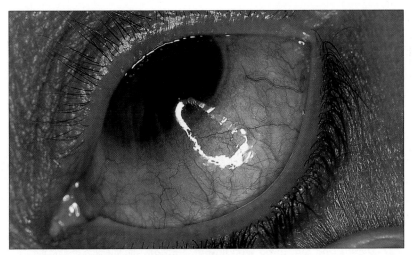

225 Episcleritis in systemic lupus erythematosus. The redness is marked at the inner limbic area, the dilated vessels lying between the conjunctiva and the sclera. There is no discharge. Usually this is segmental, covering one or two quadrants, and is often associated with rheumatoid arthritis, collagen disease, and Reiter's disease. It may be painful, but vision is not impaired.

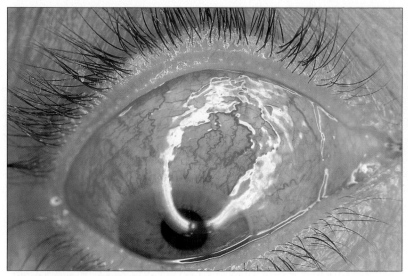

226 Dramatic episcleritis. This lady with relapsing polychondritis presented with sore, red eyes, ears and nose.

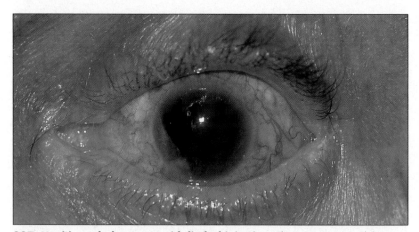

227 Uveitis and glaucoma with limbal injection. The injection around the limbus is part of the clinical picture of uveitis. In iritis, there is pain, photophobia and blurring of vision. Uveitis may be associated with systemic conditions; chronic infection like syphilis, Lyme disease and tuberculosis; parasitic disease such as toxoplasmosis; chronic granulomatous disease such as sarcoidosis; chronic inflammatory bowel disease; and collagen diseases such as ankylosing spondylitis.

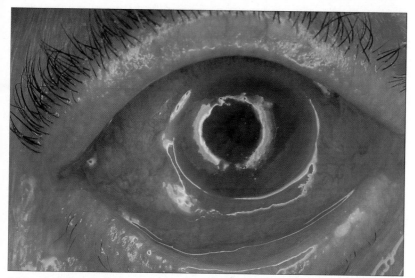

228 Absolute glaucoma. The end result of untreated acute glaucoma, leading to loss of vision.

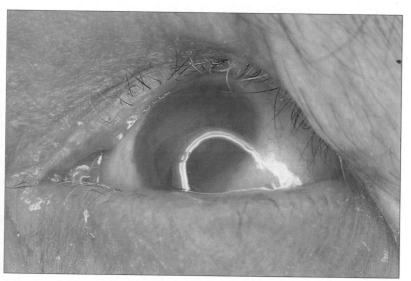

229 Corneal opacity secondary to ingrowing eyelashes and trachoma.
Upper tarsal scars from endemic trachoma lead to ingrowing eyelashes.

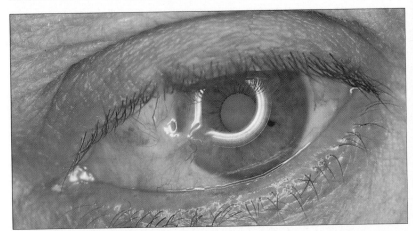

230 Cataract and pterygium. The cataract produces the white lens opacity. Early cataracts may be less obvious and be seen with the +12-dioptre lens of the opthalmoscope as central polar cataracts. Cataracts may be congenital, due to old age, secondary to trauma either physical or from ionising radiation, and may complicate diabetes mellitus, hypocalcaemia and local or systemic corticosteroid therapy. The pterygium is a benign leash of vessels and fibrous tissue, which spreads across the eye and only becomes significant if it encroaches on the cornea and interferes with vision.

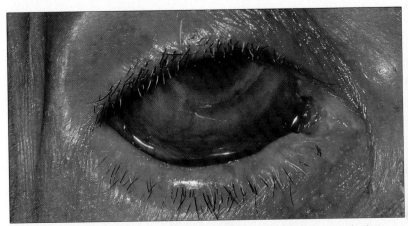

231 Argyria. This Bedouin Arab has 'black eyes.' Both the conjunctiva and sclera are affected. This eye had silver nitrate eye drops placed in it for many years as a remedy for redness associated with climatic conditions. Industrial exposure and medication with silver salts may lead to a slate-grey pigmentation of the skin or nail beds.

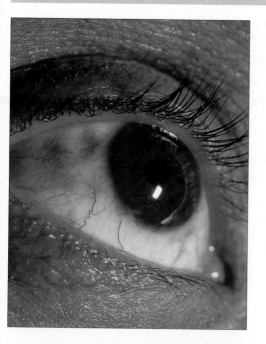

232 Racial melanosis of the conjunctiva. Brown pigmentation of the sclera may be seen in dark-skinned races.

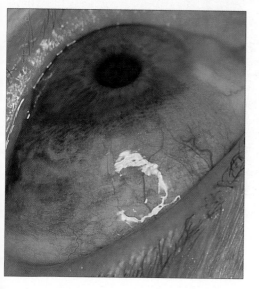

233 Melanosis of conjunctiva. This is of no significance and varies in amount. The possibility of melanoma should be considered.

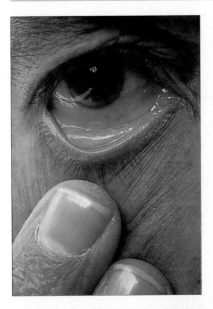

234 Yellow sclera and buffed nails indicating cholestatic jaundice. Cholestatic jaundice is deduced by examining the nails. Bilirubin stains the sclera, the tint ranging from palest lemon to deepest saffron. The whiteness of the sclera depends on the colour of the light reflected from it; daylight is best. Yellow clothes and blankets should be removed. The nails are buffed at the tips and not near the cuticle as if they have a coat of nail polish (*see* **473**)—this is **the sign of the chronic pruritic**. Pruritus may have many causes. This degree of polish has been produced by several weeks' itching. Causes of itching include liver disease even without jaundice, parasitic infestation, eczema, old age, drugs, and malignant and metabolic disease (e.g. diabetes mellitus and renal failure).

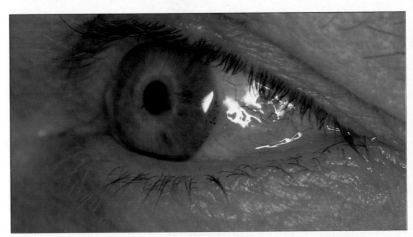

235 Limbal pigmentation in ochronosis (Alcaptonuria, *see* **267).** This man and his brother had premature degenerative joint disease. There is brown pigment deposition at the limbus and a pterygium. Brown pigment could be copper as in Wilson's disease (*see* **240**), racial (*see* **232**), due to rust from iron deposition, or due to silver deposition (*see* **231**). The brown colour may affect all the sclera. Look at the ears (*see* **264**).

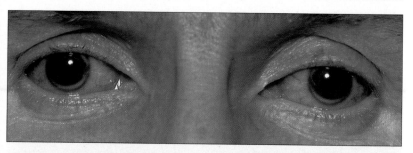

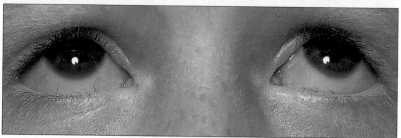

236 Blue sclera—father and son—due to type I osteogenesis imperfecta.
The juvenile arcus is common and unexplained. Lipid abnormalities are usually excluded. The blue colour reflects the thin sclera due to a reduction of collagen, which affects both skeletal and non-skeletal tissues; look for incompetent heart valves. In women, fractures may be delayed until the perimenopause and increased osteoporosis develops.

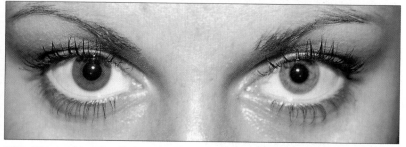

237 Heterochromia. This could be due to a right contact lens, a glass eye, Horner's syndrome from birth trauma when the iris may fail to darken, recurrent anterior uveitis or Waardenburg's syndrome.[33] But she has no ptosis, cataract, deafness or white hair.

---

[33]Petrus Johannes Waardenburg, Dutch ophthalmologist, 1886–1979. A new syndrome combining developmental anomalies of the eyelids, eyebrows, and nose root with pigmentary defects of the iris and head hair with congenital deafness autosomal dominant. *Am. J. Hum. Genet.*, 1951, **3**: 195–253.

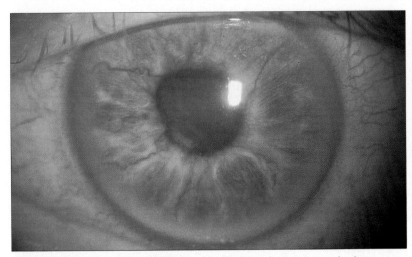

238 Rubeotic iris with an irregular pupil. Rubeotic glaucoma with ciliary injection, a hazy cornea due to oedema, new vessel formation on the iris and an irregular pupil. Neovascularisation is a response to ocular ischaemia of any cause such as diabetes mellitus, arteritis, or carotid artery disease or retinal vein thrombosis.

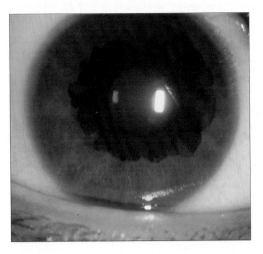

239 Iris hamartomas (Lisch nodules). These are raised pin-head nodules on the iris. They are present in over 90% of individuals with type I neurofibromatosis (NF) by the age of 20 years.[34] Their presence may allow confirmation of the diagnosis of this disease, which is inherited as an autosomal dominant with incomplete penetrance.

[34]Lubs, ML. Bauer, MS. Formas, ME. Djokic, B. Lisch nodules in NF Type I. *N. Eng. J. Med.*, 1991, **324**: 1264–6.

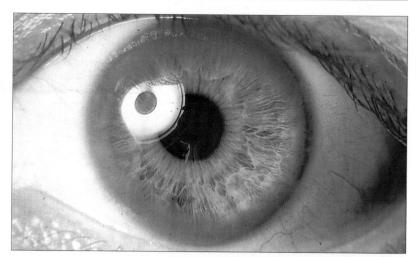

240 Kayser–Fleischer[35] ring. This starts initially as a brown rusty muddiness at 12 and 6 o'clock. Here it forms a complete rim around the cornea. It is caused by a deposition of copper in Desçemet's[36] membrane of the cornea in Wilson's[37] disease.

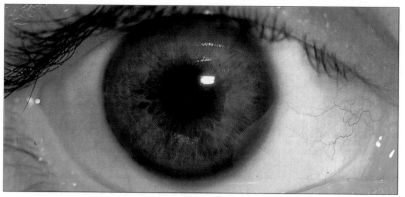

241 Kayser–Fleischer ring on a blue eye.

---

[35]Bernard Kayser, German ophthalmologist, 1869–1954. Über einen Fall von angeborener grünlicher Verfärbung de Cornea. *Klin. Mbl. Augenh.*, 1902, **40(2)**: 22–5. Bruno Fleischer, German ophthalmologist, 1848–1904. Zwei weitere Fälle von grünlicher Verfäubung der Kornea. *Klin. Mbl. Augenh.*, 1903, **41(1)**: 489–91.

[36]Jean Desçemet, French anatomist, 1732–1810.

[37]Samuel Alexander Kinnier Wilson, 1878–1936. Progressive lenticular degeneration. A familial nervous disease associated with cirrhosis of the liver. *Brain*, 1912, **34**: 295–509.

IRREGULAR PUPILS

Patients do not complain of irregular pupils, but may complain of blurred vision. When assessing unequal pupils consider whether they are regular and unequal, or irregular and unequal. If the latter there is usually a local cause. Analyse them on the basis of an **abnormal small pupil** and its possibilities, and then **an abnormal large pupil** and its possibilities. The cause will become clear.

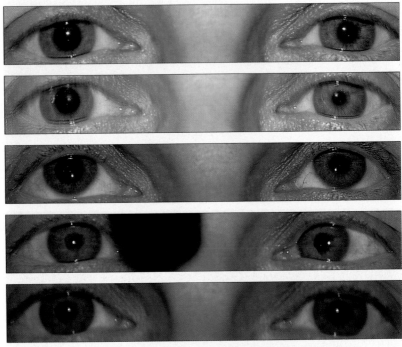

242 Unequal regular pupils (anisocoria)—Holmes Adie[38] pupils. The sequence shown is as follows: **at rest**—a tonic right pupil; the **reaction of the pupils to light**—the left constricts; **on looking up** and **on looking at a finger** (i.e. accommodation) shows light near dissociation; **at rest again**—redilation tonicity on the affected side has caused transient reversal of the inequality. Physiological inequality occurs in 20% of people. Anisocoria is usually associated with the Holmes Adie syndrome of tonic pupil with absent tendon reflexes. Other causes include trauma, syphilis, herpes zoster and temporal arteritis.

---

[38]Gordon Morgan Holmes, British neurologist, 1876–1965. William John Adie, 1886–1935. Adie, WJ. Pseudo-Argyll Robinson pupils with absent tendon reflexes. A benign disorder simulating tabes dorsalis. *Br. Med. J.*, 1931, **1**: 928–30. Holmes, G. Partial iridoplegia associated with other symptoms of the nervous system. *Tr. Ophth. Soc. U.K.*, 1931, **51**: 209–28.

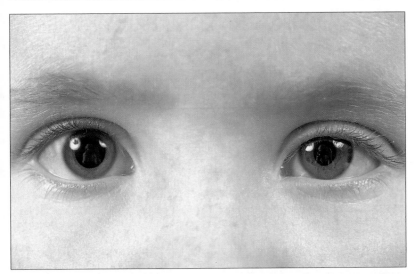

243 Unequal but regular pupil. A pharmacologically-dilated pupil using atropine tends to be larger than that of a third nerve palsy. It may be accidental or deliberate, and is commonly a contamination from a family member who has used atropine eyedrops.

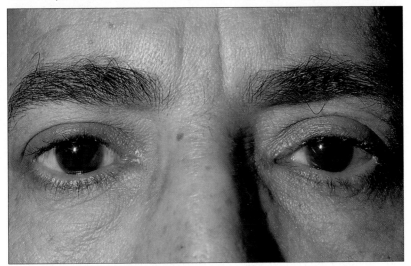

244 Constricted but equal pupils. This man smoked opium. A more common cause is the instillation of drops containing pilocarpine for glaucoma. The use of morphine or heroin will lead to tiny pupils.

Bilateral tonic or poorly reactive pupils, and those that are irregular or show light near dissociation may be due to tertiary syphilis, which should always be excluded.

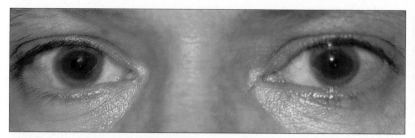

245 Unequal and irregular pupils. These small pupils react poorly to mydriatics and are associated with positive syphilis serology; they are a feature of **tabes dorsalis**.

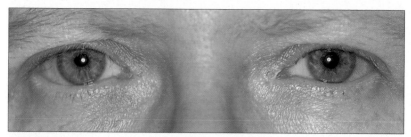

246 The classic pupil of neurosyphilis—Argyll Robertson pupils. A small irregular pupil, which reacts poorly to light, but briskly accommodates, and reacts slowly to mydriatics. There is depigmentation of the iris adjacent to the pupil.

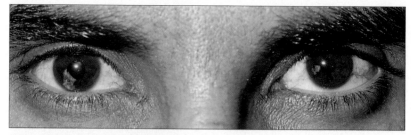

247 Unequal but regular pupils. The right pupil is larger than the left and a band of white spans the radius of the iris, but on the left the span is not complete. This is due to a failure of the circular muscle to develop completely, which is therefore weaker on the right and does not constrict well to light. This is a **coloboma of the eye.**

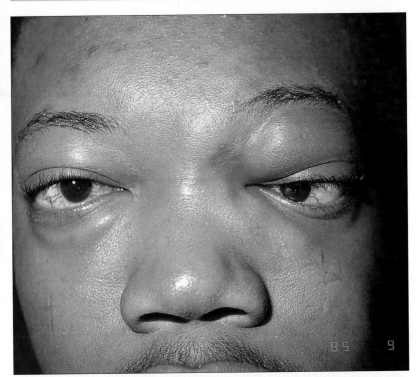

248 Carotico-cavernous fistula (CCF). A lover of very loud disco music complained of noises in his ears in bed at night! He has proptosis and conjunctival injection on both sides, reflecting a cross flow of blood. He has an oculomotor palsy due to nerve compression in the cavernous sinus. The high pressure leak from the artery to the cavernous sinus produces the bruit, which is both heard and felt. It is obliterated by ipsilateral carotid compression. A CCF may be caused by a basal skull fracture tearing the carotid artery in the sinus or by spontaneous aneurysmal rupture. Defective collagen in the Ehlers–Danlos[39] syndrome, with joint hyperextensibilty and skin fragility, may lead to visceral or arterial rupture.

---

[39]Edvard Ehlers, Danish dermatologist, 1863–1937. Ehlers, E. Neigung zu Hämorrhagien in der Haut, Lockerung mehrerer Artikulationen. *Derm. Zschr.*, 1901, **8**: 173–4. Henri Alexandre Danlos, French physician, 1844–1912. Danlos, H. Un cas de cutis laxa avec tumeurs por contusion chronique de coudes et des genoux (xanthoma juvenile pseudo-diabetique de MM.Hallopeau et Mace de Lepinay). *Bull. Soc. Fr. Derm. Syph.*, 1908, **19**: 70–2.

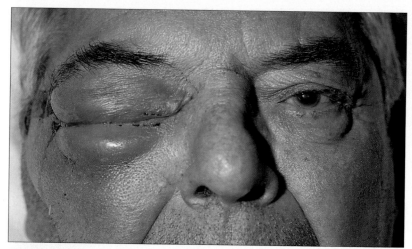

249 Erysipelas. A rigor in the night was followed by a tingling in the facial skin and 12 hours later this appearance. This man has a bacterial infection of the dermis and superficial lymphatics.

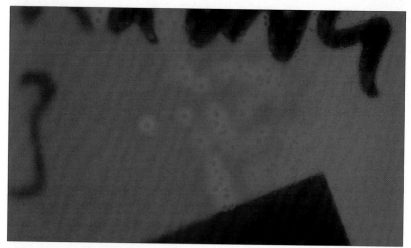

250 Culture plate of man in 249 growing haemolytic streptococci. The bacterial cause of the erysipelas was *Streptococcus pyogenes,* which shows characteristic haemolysis around the colonies. Cellulitis is a deeper infection than erysipelas and less distinct, whereas fasciitis occurs deep to fascia and damages local nutrient vessels, leading to gangrene.

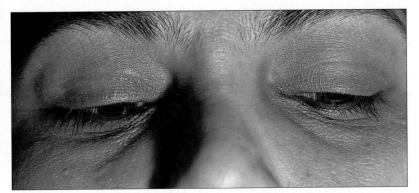

251 Lacrimal gland enlargement. The lacrimal gland can be seen peeping out at the right lateral orbital margin and may be seen in Mikulicz's[40] syndrome of salivary and lacrimal gland enlargement with xerostomia. This is most frequently due to sarcoidosis, though lymphoma, infection or leukaemia may produce the same picture.

FUNDAL PHOTOGRAPHS

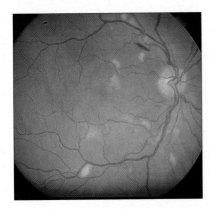

252a Cotton wool spot (CWS) stage in AIDS. This appearance represents arteriolar infarcts due to immune complex deposition in the vessel. It lasts one to six weeks. The CWS represents an accumulation of axoplasm, from the nerve fibre axons damaged by an inadequate blood supply, and later ingested by macrophages forming the cytoid body. Similar changes may occur in the vasculitis of polyarteritis nodosa and systemic lupus erythematosus. CWS may be seen in hypertension, diabetes mellitus, retinal vein occlusion, microemboli, acute pancreatitis and other vasculitides.

---

[40]Mikulicz, J. Polish surgeon, 1850–1905. Über eine eigenartige symmetrische Erkrankung der Träuenund Mundspeicheldrusen. *Beitr. Chir. Fortschr.* Gewidmet Theodor Billroth, Stuttgart, 1892, pp. 610–30.

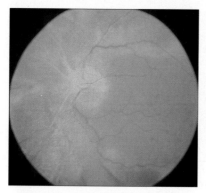

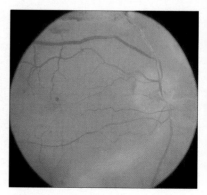

252b Retinal infiltrates in AIDS. This cellular infiltrate is due to cytomegalovirus retinitis and may appear anywhere in the retina. It has a soft cheesy appearance.

252c Retinal infiltrates in AIDS. There are some retinal haemorrhages.

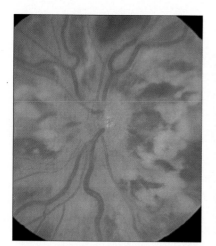

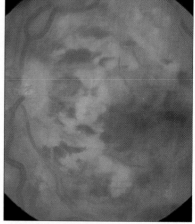

253 Central retinal vein thrombosis. The 'blood storm' appearance centred on the disc (left) and the macular (right). Note a blotch haemorrhage at the top left and extensive diffuse haemorrhage and cotton wool spots. A branch vein occlusion has these changes limited to a segment of retina. Retinal vein thrombosis may be more frequent with age and complicate diabetes mellitus, hypertension, polycythaemia, macroglobulinaemia, glaucoma and systemic inflammation. Subsequent vascularisation may occur—rubeosis iridis (*see* **238**).

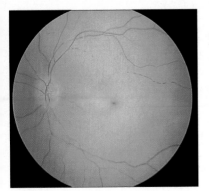

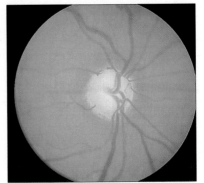

254 Central retinal artery occlusion.

Sudden painless loss of vision in one eye and an afferent pupillary defect. Arterial occlusion (usually embolic) leads to the 'cattle trucking' appearance with empty gaps in the blood column. Emboli may be seen as yellow or grey cholesterol fragments. There is cloudy swelling of the ganglion and nerve fibre cell layers producing the milky white colour of the retina. If an arterial branch only is affected, then the changes are limited to that segment and there is a segmental visual field defect. Ultimately there is optic nerve atrophy. The cherry red spot is due to the normal choroidal red reflex showing though the gap at the fovea where the ganglion cells and nerve fibre layer are pushed aside. This is also seen in Tay–Sachs[41] disease where gangliosides are deposited in the retinal ganglion cells and obscure the normal colour which shows through at the fovea. The differential diagnosis of painless sudden loss of vision in one eye is retrobulbar neuritis, ischaemic optic neuritis, central retinal artery occlusion, vitreous haemorrhage and a retinal detachment.

255 Primary optic atrophy.

Dramatic pallor of the disc with a defined edge and loss of direct reaction of the pupil to light, a central scotoma may be present. The end result of an insult to the nerve head and develops after neuritis, nerve compression, or ischaemia. Relative afferent pupillary defects on light stimulation occur in central retinal artery occlusion, ischaemic optic neuropathy (cranial arteritis), optic neuritis, retinal detachment, unilateral glaucoma and optic nerve compression.

[41]Warren Tay, British physician, 1843–1927. Symmetrical changes in the region of the yellow spot in each eye of an infant. Tr. Opth. Soc. U.K., 1881,**1**:57–7
Bernard Sachs, US physician, 1858–1944. On arrested cerebral development, with special reference to its cortical pathology. J. Nerv. Ment. Dis., 1887, **14**:541–53.

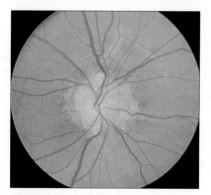

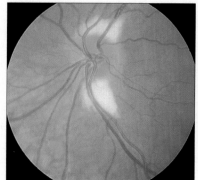

256a Optic disc drusen. Buried hyaline bodies produce the drusen at the disc—an appearance of pseudo-papilloedema. Remember that if spontaneous retinal vein pulsation is present (it may be absent in 20% of normal people but brought out by gentle pressure on the globe), then papilloedema is unlikely. Angioid streaks are present radiating as red lines from the disc edge and represent anatomical defects in Bruch's membrane—and are also seen in pseudoxanthoma elasticum, Ehlers–Danlos syndrome and sickle cell disease.

256b Myelinated nerve fibres. White patches with a feathery margin. The fibres of the optic nerve lose their myelin sheath on entering the eye. If it persists after the fibres leave the disc, it may obscure both vessels and disc.

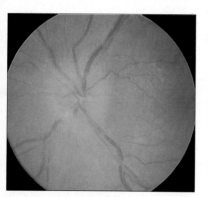

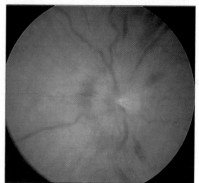

257a Papilloedema. The edge of the optic disc is blurred and heaped up. Swelling of the optic nerve head is secondary to raised intracranial pressure (ICP). Disc oedema occurs without raised ICP as a secondary change in optic papillitis, ischaemic optic neuropathy, central retinal vein occlusion and hypertension. Drusen and hypermetropia should be excluded.

257b Malignant hypertension. Papilloedema with a blurred swollen disc surrounded by oedematous retina and exudates (macular star) may precipitate in the superficial retina. There is arterial narrowing, arteriovenous nipping superiorly and flame-shaped haemorrhages in accelerated hypertension.

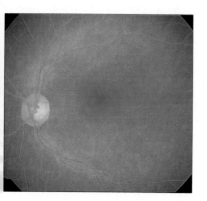

258 Lipaemia retinalis. Orange rather than red vessels due to the presence of fat in hypertriglyceridaemia. It may be seen in poorly controlled diabetics.

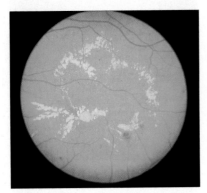

259a Diabetic retinopathy. Circinate
retinopathy with hard exudates encircling
the macula. Plasma leaks from the vessels
and lipoprotein is taken up by macrophages
and appears as hard exudates. The circular
distribution of the exudates defines the
junction of normal and abnormal retina.
There are scattered microaneurysms.

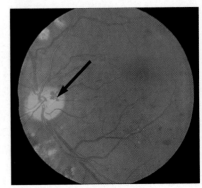

259b Diabetic retinopathy.
Neovascularisation in response to
ischaemia. At the disc abnormal
capillaries have budded and formed a tuft
of vessels which are prone to bleeding,
the vessels will bring with them fibrous
tissue which can contract and pull on the
retina.

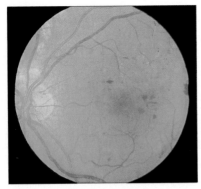

259c Diabetic retinopathy.
Microaneurysms–small red round
dots–represent herniated endothelial cell
proliferation through the abnormal capillary
wall. There is retinal new vessel formation.

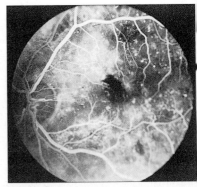

259d Diabetic retinopathy. The
fluorescein angiogram shows hyper-
fluorescence due to leakage through the
abnormal capillary wall of fats and proteins
into the retina. Microaneurysms are seen as
white dots.

The ear

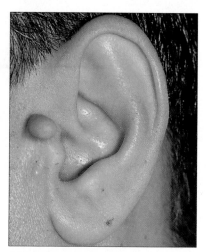

260 Accessory auricle.
Hillocks or accessory lobules found anterior to the tragus may require excision for cosmetic reasons.

261 Pre-auricular sinus. This is a remnant of the branchial cleft. It may get infected. The opening of the sinus is difficult to see and is the clue to the cause of inflammation on the other side.

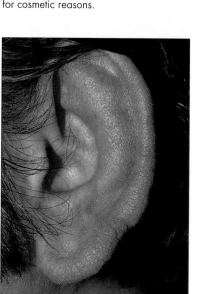

262 Haemangioma on the pinna.
The cavernous vascular malformation produces thickening of the ear, and a change in colour and texture, which also involves the skin on the neck. Compare this with the ear of lepromatous leprosy (*see* **121**).

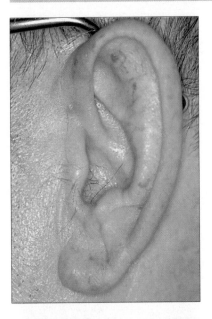

263 Hereditary haemorrhagic telangiectasia. The ear is a common site to see dilated capillary loops (*see* **46**).

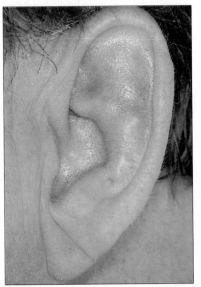

264 Ochronosis—grey ears. This is inherited as an autosomal recessive disorder. Decreased activity of homogentisate oxidase leads to an accumulation of homogentisic acid, pigmentation (first described microscopically by Virchow[41] as ochronosis as in ochre) and premature degeneration of cartilage. This leads to the grey colour showing through from the darkened cartilage. The sclera may be pigmented (*see* **235**).

[42]Rudolph Ludwig Karl Virchow, German pathologist, 1821–1902.

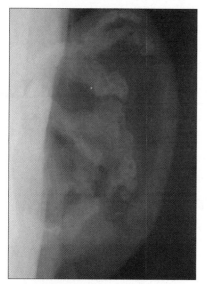

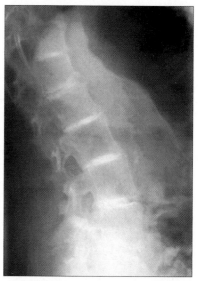

265 Ochronosis of the pinna (radiograph). Calcification is obvious in the rigid ear cartilage. Chondrocalcinosis may occur after trauma (the cauliflower ear) and in joint cartilage in gout, pseudogout, osteoarthritis and diseases involving divalent metals—copper, iron, calcium. These latter diseases—Wilson's disease, haemochromatosis and hyperparathyroidism—are associated with an arthropathy.

266 Calcified intervertebral discs in ochronosis (radiograph). Progressive arthritis is a feature of ochronosis and particularly affects the spine.

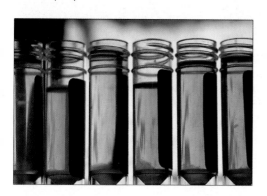

267 Alkaptonuria. A day's urine specimens—the oldest urine is on the right. Darkening of the urine on standing is due to oxidation of homogentisic acid. It may give false positive tests for sugar unless a glucose oxidase method is used (dipstix rather than tablets).

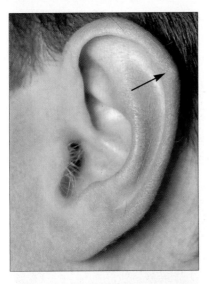

268 Darwin's[42] tubercle. This tubercle, equivalent to the pointed tip of the ear seen in many mammals, has the eponym of the Naturalist's name and should not be confused with a gouty tophus (*see* **269, 270**)

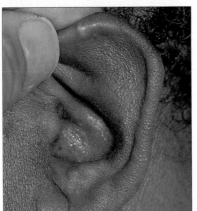

269 A gouty tophus. This is due to the deposition of sodium urate in the cartilage and transmits a characteristic ivory tint through the skin.

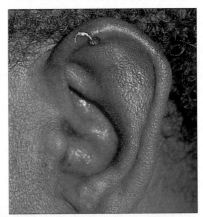

270 Urate squeezed from the tophus. The sodium urate will ooze out like toothpaste if punctured. Demonstration of urate crystals in joint fluid will confirm the diagnosis of acute gout, which is otherwise a clinical guess.

---

[43]Charles Darwin, naturalist, 1809–1882. *The Origin of the Species*, 24 Nov. 1859. First edition of 1250 copies all sold out that day!

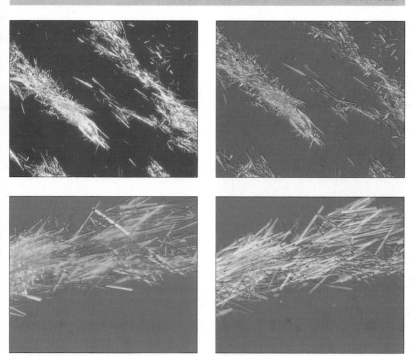

271 Urate crystals in joint fluid. On New Year's Eve a man presented with a five-day history of severe pain in his right wrist, said to be due to a fall in the last few days, which he could not remember! The joint was aspirated and the fluid viewed by light passing through two crossed polarisers (top left and top right with the addition of a red filter)—the crystals are visible because they can split the polarised ray due to the property of birefringence. A first-order red filter is inserted at 0°(bottom left) and turned by 90° rotation (bottom right) and demonstrates that the crystals are also dichroic. The diagnosis of acute gout was confirmed and the patient improved on appropriate treatment. The only definitive test to prove that an acute monoarthritis is acute gout is for the urate crystal to be viewed through two polarisers at right angles to each other.The crystal demonstrates the property of birefringence in that it splits the polarised light into two part rays, which are refracted along different paths. If a first-order red filter is then inserted and viewed at 0° and then when turned through 90°, two different colours appear. The change in colour is due to differential absorption of light depending upon the direction of vibration of the part rays in a birefringent substance. The crystal is dichroic.

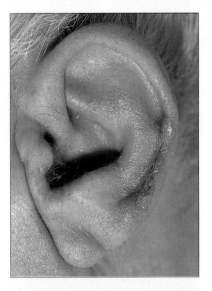

272 Transverse ear lobe crease (ELC) and solar keratosis of the pinna. The transverse ELC is more common in middle age (see **264**). An association with ischaemic heart disease could reflect the confounding effect of age and obesity, but a review of risk factors is prudent[44]. A **solar keratosis** is the area of adherent hyperkeratosis on the helix—a common site in men—due to the cumulative effect of sunlight on exposed skin. It may be pre-malignant.

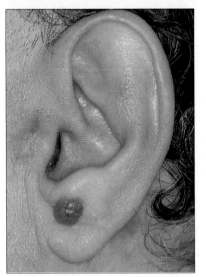

273 Cautery to treat Bell's palsy. A Bedouin from the desert of Arabia with a recovering lower motor neurone facial palsy and a fresh burn scar adjacent to the tragus—a common therapy for disease. Since 80% of Bell's palsies recover spontaneously, the cautery has an 80% cure rate!

---

[44]Physical signs should be prompts to further thought and not be taken as concrete evidence. Patel *et al.* Diagonal ear lobe creases and atheromatous disease: a post-mortem study. *J. Roy. Coll. Phys.* (Lond.), 1992, **26(3)**: 274–7.

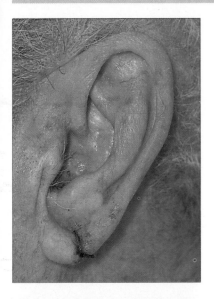

274 Slit to the ear to treat a stroke. A Greek Cypriot in Holloway London was treated by his daughter with blood letting for his sudden right-sided hemiplegia. She opened the ear lobe with a razor blade. This is a folk remedy for 'stroke', particularly in the Mediterranean area.[45]

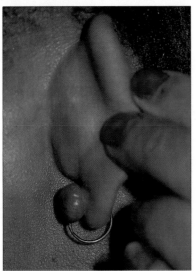

275 Keloid on the back of the ear lobe—why on the back? The ear is a common site for keloid formation, often on the inside of the lobe, which could reflect the direction of piercing.

---

[45]William Osler, *The Principles and Practice of Medicine,* 1st ed., 1892, p. 882. Treatment of cerebral haemorrhage "most satisfactory is venesection…whenever the arterial tension is much increased."

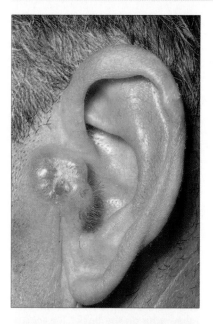

276 Basal cell carcinoma ear.
There is a ulcer with central
hyperkeratosis in the pre-auricular area.
Bleeding points are revealed when the
crust is removed. The ulcer shows
peripheral telangiectasia and has a raised
rolled margin. There is a solar keratosis
on the helix.

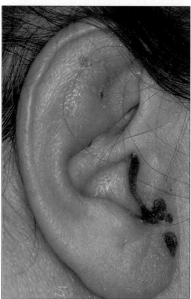

**277 Ramsay Hunt syndrome—
herpes zoster ear.** This is a pointer to
the cause of a lower motor neurone facial
palsy. Herpes zoster affecting the
geniculate ganglion produces herpetic
vesicles around the external auditory
meatus and on the soft palate.

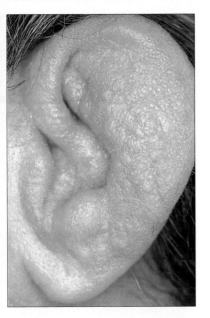

278 Relapsing polychondritis. Two weeks with a hoarse voice and pain in the ears, eyes and nose led to consultation. The pinna and tragus are tender, red and swollen, but the lobe is spared; only the cartilage-containing parts are inflamed.

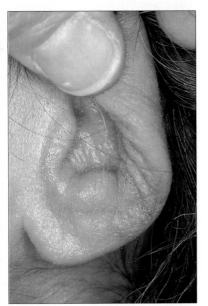

279 Relapsing polychondritis. When the pinna is folded forwards it rolls up like wet felt. There was intense scleritis (*see* **226**) and the nose was deformed (*see* **281**).

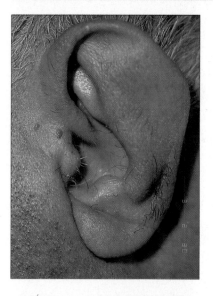

280 Relapsing polychondritis. The illness of the patient shown in **278** and **279** relapsed and remitted, leaving the pinna without cartilaginous support 10 years later.

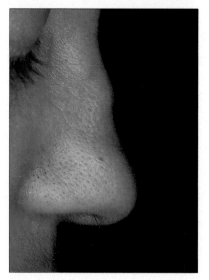

281 Nasal cartilage in relapsing polychondritis. Deformity of the nose may affect the cartilage or the bony bridge. In relapsing polychondritis, the cartilage softens, but more commonly may reflect damage from trauma, surgery, Wegener's granulomatosis[46] and tumour infiltration. If the depression is in the bony part then congenital syphilis or midline tumours are possibilities.

---

[46]Friedrich Wegener, German pathologist, born 1907. Über eine eigenartige rhinogene Granulomatose mit besonderer Beteiligung des Arteriensystems und Nieren. *Beitr. Path. Anat.*, 1939, **102**: 36–68.

THE MOUTH

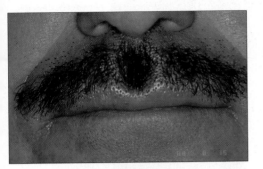

282 A swollen lip. An elderly man with a swollen itchy lip. Trauma, angioedema and drug allergy were excluded. This is hypersensitivity to phenylenediamine in black moustache dye!

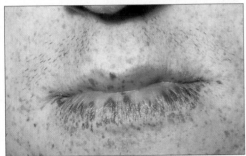

283 Peutz–Jeghers[47] syndrome (the lips). Circumoral and mucosal pigmented macules in the mouth and on the face, often more on the lower lip, are inherited as an autosomal dominant gene. Associated gastrointestinal polyposis affects the upper gastro-intestinal tract more than the colon. Malignant change is commoner in the upper gastrointestinal tract. Macules may be seen on the hands, feet and nails.

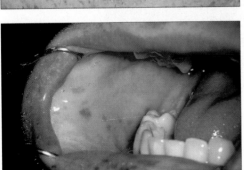

284 Peutz–Jeghers macules on the buccal mucosa. The macules must be differentiated from the more diffuse pigmentation of Addison's disease (*see* **30, 31**).

---

[47]JLA Peutz, Dutch physician. Peutz, JLA. Over een zeer merkvaardige, gecombinerde familiaire polyposis van de slijmvliezen, van den tractus intestinalis met die van de neuskeelholte en gepaard met eigen-aardige pigmentaties van huiden slijmvliezen. *Ned. Mschr. Genesk.*, 1921, **10**: 134–46.

Harold Joseph Jeghers, American physician, born 1904. Jeghers H. *et al.* Generalised intestinal poly-posis and melanin spots on the oral mucosa, lips and digits. A syndrome of diagnostic significance. *N. Eng. J. Med.*, 1949, **241**: 993–1005.

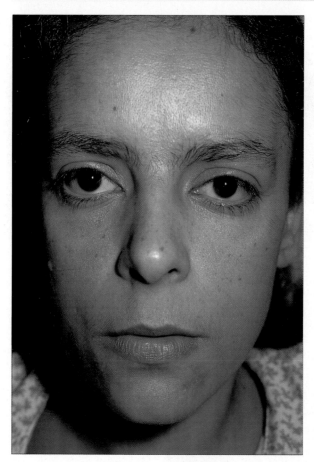

285 The cyanosed mouth. The lips have the blue tint of cyanosis,[48] which requires the presence of more than 5 g/dl of reduced haemoglobin. Look at the tongue. Peripheral cyanosis is due to a slowing of flow and increased extraction of oxygen. Central cyanosis may be due to reduced arterial oxygen saturation or the presence of an abnormal haemoglobin.

---

[48]In the Caucasian, cyanosis can be detected when oxygen saturation is reduced to 85%, but in a dark-skinned person, it may not be apparent until it falls to 75%. There must be an increase in total venous blood in the skin or a fall in oxygen saturation. It is apparent when the mean capillary concentration of reduced haemoglobin exceeds 5 g/dl. The absolute value rather than the relative value is what is important, for in anaemia there may be marked desaturation and yet no cyanosis is seen. In polycythaemia, cyanosis may be apparent at higher levels of saturation.,

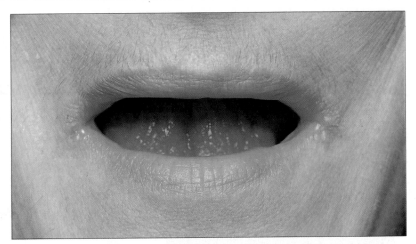

286 Angular cheilitis. A complaint of soreness of the angles of the mouth. Sore corners, cracking and some inflammation is often blamed on diet or candidiasis. The teeth are absent. As the gums shrink, the mandibular bone is reabsorbed, the jaws overclose, and the angles of the mouth become opposed producing a moist soggy area prone to maceration and secondary infection. New denture linings will open the bite and may heal the angles of the mouth.

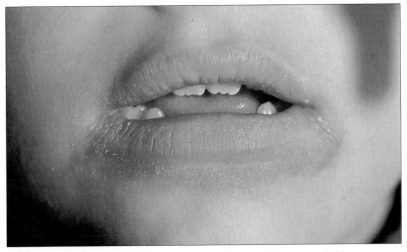

287 Lick eczema secondarily infected with *Candida*. Young children may become habitual lickers and smackers, the area of soreness reflecting the lip licking.

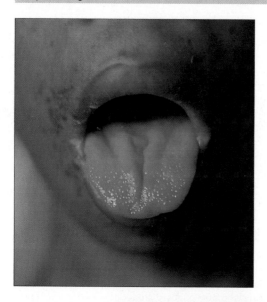

288 Angular cheilosis, glossitis and skin scaling. This malnourished individual had a smooth red tongue, glossitis, angular soreness and pigmented desquamation.

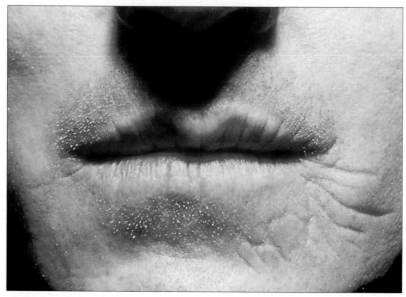

289 Rhagades. The acute rhagades that radiate from the mouth in congenital syphilis are, unlike malnutrition, less inflamed and heal with scarring.

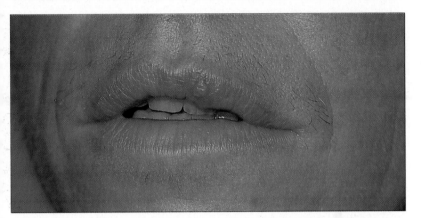

290 Herpes labialis—the cold sore. Recurrent herpes simplex virus 1 frequently affects the lip and differs from primary herpes simplex virus infection by the lack of systemic upset and resolution in 6–7 days. Recurrence seems to be associated with trauma, febrile illnesses, exposure to sunlight, surgery and stress. It may precede recurrent erythema multiforme by several days.

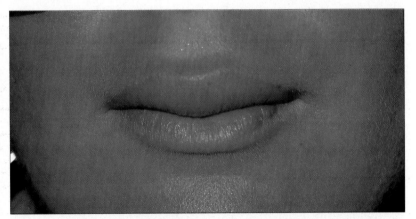

291 The swollen lip (macrocheilia) due to angioedema. Sudden swelling of the lips may be traumatic, due to allergy or urticaria, or related to C1-esterase inhibitor deficiency as in hereditary angioedema. A more chronic presentation may be due to a developmental, infective or acquired granulomatous condition such as sarcoidosis and Crohn's[49] disease.

---

[49]Bernard Burril Crohn, American gastroenterologist, 1884–1983. Regional ileitis—a pathologic and clinical entity. *J. A. M. A.*, 1932, **99**: 1323–9.

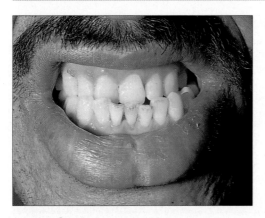

292 Macrochelia (fat lips). The increase in soft tissue makes the lips succulent and this is magnified by the prognathic mandibular overbite. Increased growth hormone in **acromegaly** leads to overgrowth of soft tissue.

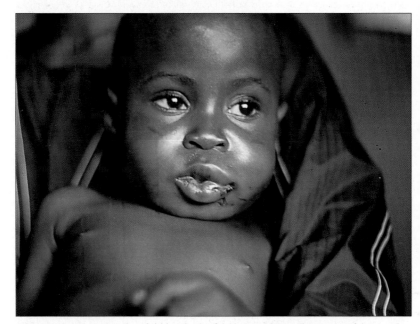

293 Cancrum oris. This child has had a febrile convulsion. The corner of the mouth has been torn by the insertion of a wooden gag at the time of the convulsion. The cheek is swollen because the inner aspect is necrotic following a breakdown in mucosal integrity and anaerobic infection. Cancrum oris is common in Africa and is often a sequel to exanthemata in small children who are protein–calorie malnourished, ill and become dehydrated.

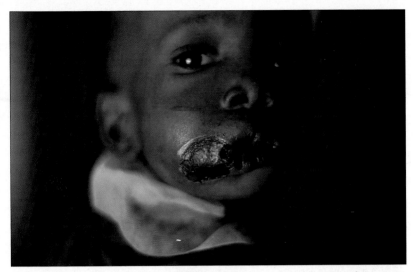

294 Cancrum oris and gangrene. The condition progresses rapidly to full thickness necrosis and sloughing (*see* **295**).

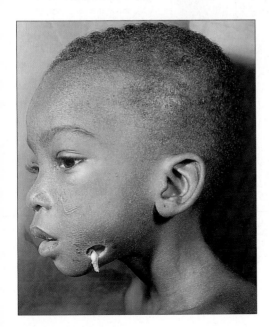

295 Cancrum oris and sloughing. While this is rare in developed countries, it may complicate the course in terminally ill, immunosuppressed patients.

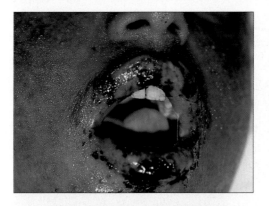

296 Haemorrhagic crusting of the lips. Mucosal ulceration and haemorrhagic crusting may be drug-induced and is a feature of the Stevens–Johnson[50] syndrome, which is often due to drugs.

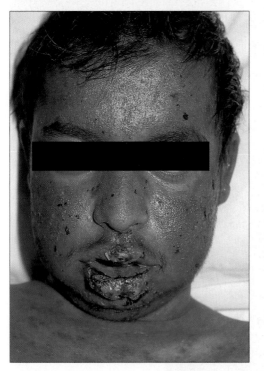

297 Stevens–Johnson syndrome (erythema multiforme). Erythema multiforme is a reaction pattern to many different stimuli ranging from herpes simplex and human immunodeficiency virus through to mycoplasma and a variety of infections, autoimmune disease and drugs. It may recur. Characteristic skin lesions may occur on the face and distal limbs (*see* **381, 841, 842**). The severe bullous form with a dramatic systemic upset and involvement of the mucous membranes, eyes and genitalia was described by Stevens and Johnson.

---

[50]Albert Mason Stevens, American physician, 1884–1945. Frank Craig Johnson, American paediatrician, 1894–1934. Stevens AM, Johnson FC., A new eruptive fever associated with stomatitis and ophthalmia. Report of two cases in children. *Am. J. Dis. Child.*, 1922, **24**: 526–33.

Swelling of the salivary glands

Swelling of the salivary glands may complicate viral infections or a chronic granulomatous disease. It may be due to a tumour.

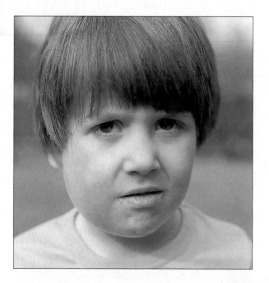

298 Unilateral facial swelling. A short history suggests an inflammatory cause, which may be viral (e.g. mumps) or bacterial causing parotitis. Intermittent swelling suggests a calculus, and long-standing swelling, a tumour. Parotid swelling in a child is usually due to mumps.

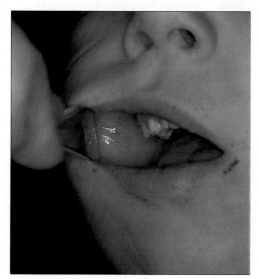

299 Parotid orifice in mumps. The inflamed parotid orifice can be see inside the mouth. In an adult mumps may be more severe with a systemic illness, abdominal and testicular pain, and headache due to meningeal involvement. In debilitated people with bacterial parotitis a drop of pus may appear at the parotid orifice.

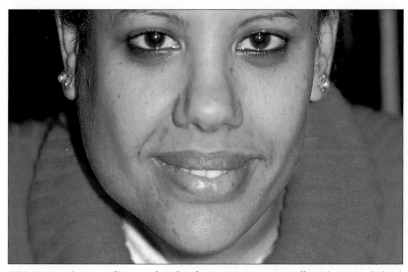

300 Intermittent salivary gland enlargement. Here, it affects the parotid gland and is due to a salivary calculus. The swelling is due to retained saliva and inflammation.

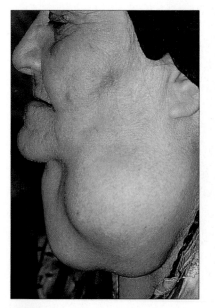

301 Submandibular enlargement. Long-standing submandibular salivary gland enlargement is usually due to a tumour or infiltration.

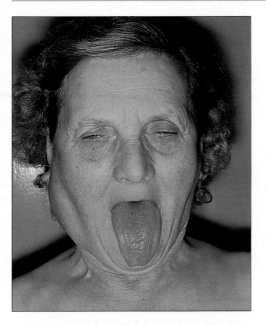

302 A dry tongue and parotid swelling. The combination of a dry tongue and dry eyes with a connective tissue disease is **Sjögren's syndrome,**[51] and the sicca or primary Sjögren's syndrome when no other disease coexists. Sjögren's syndrome is seen with sarcoidosis, collagen diseases and primary biliary cirrhosis. Other exocrine glands may be affected.

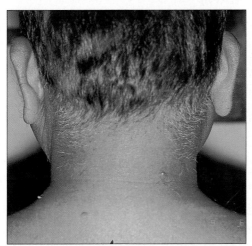

303 Long-standing bilateral glandular enlargement. "The parotids are big only if they can be seen from behind!", said a surgeon! This suggests infiltration, which can occur with lymphoma, sarcoidosis or, as here, **amyloidosis**. The parotids may be enlarged in eating disorders such as Bulimia nervosa.

---

[51]Henrik Samuel Conrad Sjögren, Swedish ophthalmologist, 1899–1986. Sjögren HS, Zur Kenntnis der Keratoconjunctivitis sicca (Keratitis filiformis bei Hypofuncktion der tränendrüsen). *Acta Ophth.* (Copenhagen), 1933, **Suppl.2**: 1–151.

Teeth and gums

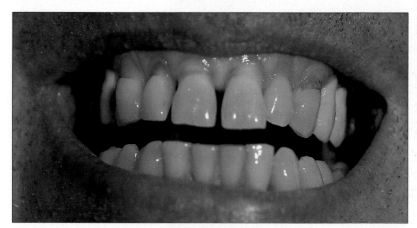

304 Tooth brush abrasion and gum recession. A disciplined childhood and the ritual of teeth cleaning produces the sign of the dominant hand and the clue to the dominant hemisphere—the right! Maximal pressure is exerted on the furthest side of the jaw away from the hand holding the brush, cutting a deep notch into his right upper canine.

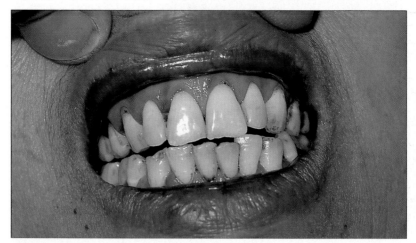

305 Chewing of a plant root for teeth cleaning. Discoloured gums may be related to pigment changes in the tissue, but may be due to substances chewed or used to clean the teeth. This man chewed on a fibrous root regularly after food.

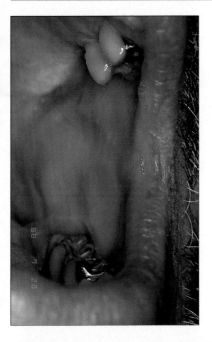

306 An assessment of financial status by examination of the mouth. Mercury amalgam fillings in the upper jaw are cheap and effective, gold inlays in the lower jaw are expensive, but long lasting. This man was a successful business man and was having his dental work upgraded—financial status going up!

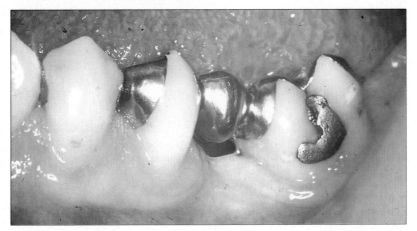

307 Gold dental inlays to the lower jaw. This precise gold work is marred by the unskilled mercury filling slapped on beside it. The creator of the inlay would not have left such a eyesore and so it must have been applied later. Perhaps the original cost bankrupted the man—financial status going down!

145

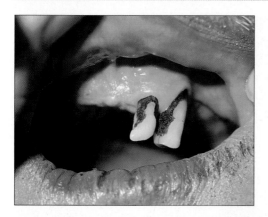

308 Body mass index of 39 kg/m² and only two teeth. Even though teeth are needed to masticate the food, their absence did not stop this man keeping his weight steady by using his thumb to push food against his teeth.

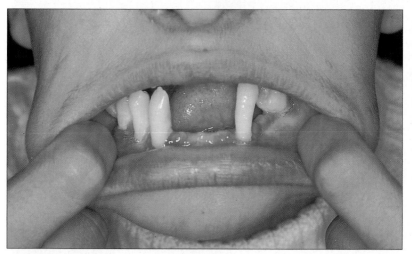

309 Gum recession. Age, plaque deposition, infection and poor tooth-cleaning technique may all lead to periodontal disease and inflammation. This causes gum recession followed by bone resorption and loosening of the teeth, the cycle culminating in loss of teeth in middle age. Here a rare cause of dental loss from periodontal disease in youth is associated with hyperkeratosis of the palms and soles—the **Papillon–Lefèvre[52] syndrome**, an autosomal recessive condition.

[52]Paul Lefèvre and Maurice Papillon, French dermatologists. Papillon M, Lefèvre P, Deux cas de keratodermie palmaire et plantaire symétrique familiale (maladie de Meleda) chez le frère et la soeur. Coexistence dans les deux cas d'alterations dentaires graves. *Bull. Soc..Fr..Derm..Syph.*, 1924, **31**: 82–7.

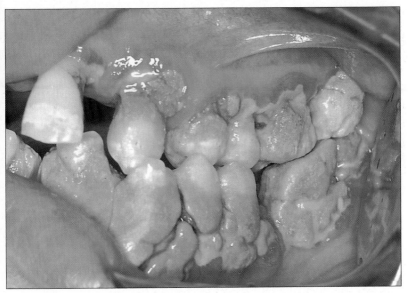

310 Dental plaque! Plaque deposition on the teeth takes 24 hours to consolidate and is usually easily removed. This vagrant has extensive plaque and calculus formation, periodontal inflammation, gum oedema and recession with loosening of the teeth.

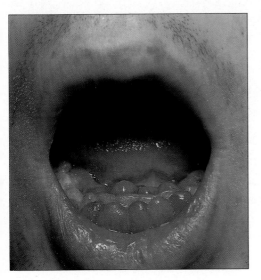

311 Gum hypertrophy.
The commonest cause of gum hypertrophy is related to poor dental hygiene. Drugs like phenytoin, nifedipine, diltiazem and cyclosporin, aggravated by poor hygiene, initially produce enlargement of the interdental papilla by stimulating fibroblasts. Blood dyscrasias may cause hypertrophy and the hormonal changes of pregnancy lead to an exaggerated inflammatory reaction to plaque and the appearance of a pyogenic granuloma or epulis.

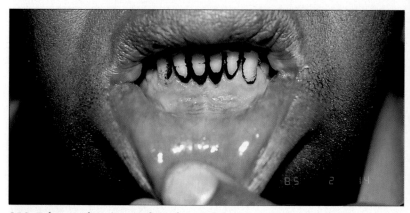

312 Tobacco chewing and tooth staining. A similar appearance may be seen with other chewing habits. The nicotine is absorbed directly into the systemic circulation, avoiding the first-pass degradation through the portal system, which would occur if the nicotine were swallowed. There is an increased incidence of oral cancer in tobacco chewers. This is **leukoplakia**. Scraping does not remove these white patches, which have developed where the wad of chewing tobacco is retained. There are many causes producing a spectrum of changes from keratosis to frank premalignant epithelial atypia. Physical and chemical irritation is common from tobacco—either smoked or chewed.

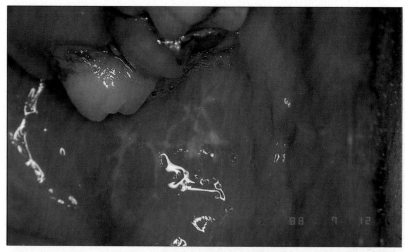

313 Frictional leukoplakia along the line of occlusion on the inside of the cheek. Friction from the teeth or denture produces frictional keratosis.

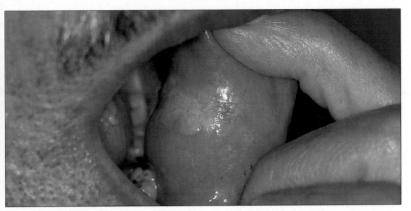

314 Leukoplakia of the inner cheek. Infections—acquired immune deficiency syndrome (AIDS), syphilis, candidiasis—are other causes, but often no cause is found.

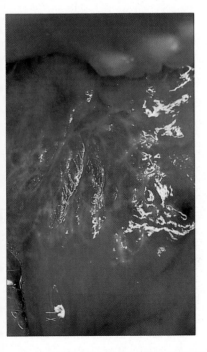

315 Oral lichen planus. White striae in a lace-like pattern (Wickham's[53] striae) and papules affect the buccal mucosa, lips or tongue. The erosive form may be painful (*see* **347**). In the mouth it must be differentiated from leukoplakia. Skin lesions are shown in **677**, **734**, **794**, **818**, **819**.

[53] Louis Frédéric Wickham, French dermatologist, 1861–1913.

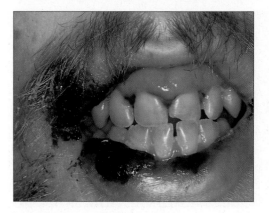

316 Bleeding of the gums. Blood oozes from the swollen interdentate papillae. Herpes simplex is present on the lips, suggesting immunosuppression. The gums that bleed with tooth brushing reflect periodontal disease, but scurvy, leukaemia and coagulation disorders must be considered.

Tooth deformity

This may be produced by:

- Interference during development from drugs.
- Chemicals and infections.
- By pressure as displacement in thumb sucking.
- By grinding in eating hard foods or for cosmetic reasons.
- From the local contact of liquids and powders.

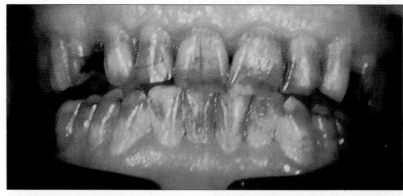

317 Discoloured teeth. The enamel is pitted and discoloured due to **fluorosis** from a naturally-occurring high fluoride level in the local water. The fluoride has been incorporated into the enamel, staining it while increasing resistance to caries. Nicotine staining can be scraped off.

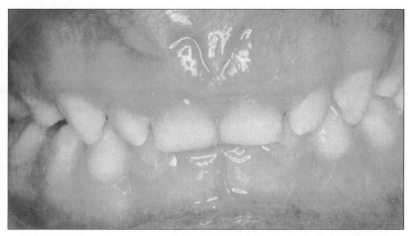

318 Tetracycline. The ingestion of tetracycline while the enamel is being laid down produces a characteristic discoloration.

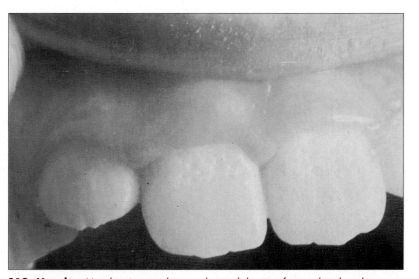

319 Measles. Measles virus produces a changed density of enamel and marks enamel formed at the time of the illness—analogous to the growth arrest lines (Beau's[54] lines) that may be seen in the nails (*see* **505, 506**).

---

[54]Honoré Simon Beau, French physician, 1806–1865. Growth arrest lines in the nails. 1846 q.v.

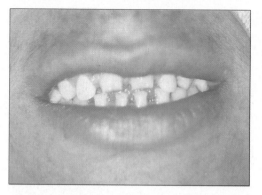

320 Hutchinson's[55] incisors. Spirochaete infection in congenital syphilis results in deformity and suppression of the middle of the three denticles from which the tooth develops. The lateral two expand unsuccessfully to fill the gap. The incisors are smaller, widely spaced, and have rounded or converging sides—screwdriver teeth. This young girl has her left eye bandaged following corneal grafting for interstitial keratitis. She has normal hearing. Hutchinson's triad[56] in congenital syphilis includes screwdriver teeth, blindness and deafness.

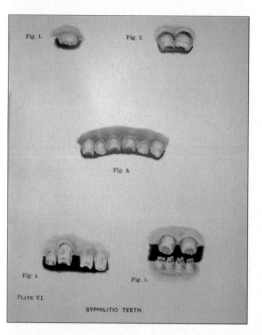

321 Hutchinson's teeth. The original illustration of Hutchison's teeth showing the different appearances depending on the state of wear of the teeth. (*Syphilis*, J. Hutchison, 1887.)

---

[55]Sir Jonathan Hutchinson, Quaker, surgeon the London Hospital, holding posts in different specialties, 1828–1913. At the end of his life persuasively promoted the idea that leprosy was caused by eating rotten fish. Hutchinson J. Report on the effects of infantile syphilis in marring the development of the teeth. *Tr. Path. Soc.* (London), 1858, **9**: 449–55.

[56]Hutchinson J. On the different forms of inflammation of the eye consequent to inherited syphilis. *Oph. Hosp. Rep.*, 1858, **1**: 191–203, 26–44; 1859, **2**: 54–105; 1860, **3**: 258–83.

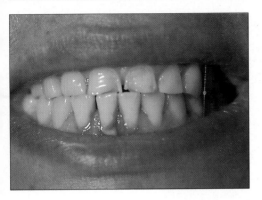

322 Dental enamel erosion. This woman weighed 125 kg (BMI 48 kg/m²) and she was advised to diet. A green salad was popular when flavoured with a lemon juice dressing. She drank a litre of it daily and the acid eroded the tooth enamel. An identical appearance may be seen when cocaine is rubbed into the gums or sniffed into the nose and mixes with the saliva. Cocaine is extracted from the leaf of the evergreen *Erythroxylum coca* with an organic solvent and then with hydrochloric acid to produce cocaine hydrochloride, which mixes with saliva to become a strong acid with a pH of 4.5. This is able to dissolve the dental mineral calcium phosphate hydroxyapatite[57]. In Bulimia nervosa, self-induced vomiting may lead to erosion of dental enamel by the gastric juices.

Inside the mouth

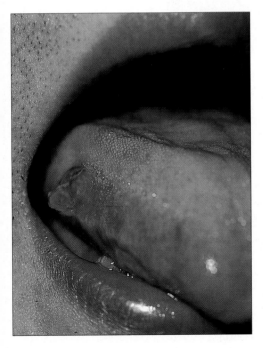

323 The bitten tongue. A traumatic mouth ulcer. He came to a casualty department confused and lethargic, with a sore tongue. He was sent home with a label of flu. The significance of his bitten tongue—a grand mal seizure—was not recognised. The diagnosis of viral encephalitis was not made until he had two more seizures.

---

[57]Krutchkoff *et al.* Cocaine induced dental erosions. *N. Eng. J. Med.*, 1990, **322(6)**: 1408.

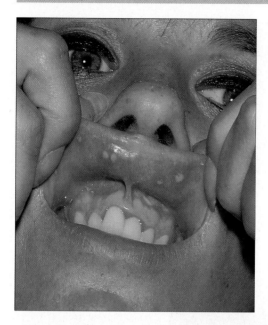

324 The recurrent ulcer.
This is common occurring in
10–30% of individuals. The
cause is unknown. In females,
minor aphthae often coincide
with the menstrual period.

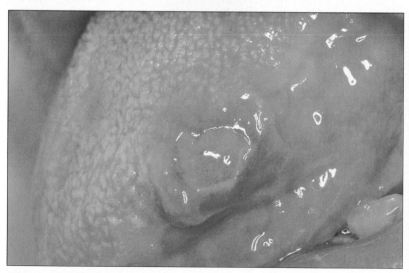

325 A minor aphthous ulcer. This is painful, with a yellow floor and a raised
erythematosus edge, and lasts 4–10 days. Other causes include trauma.

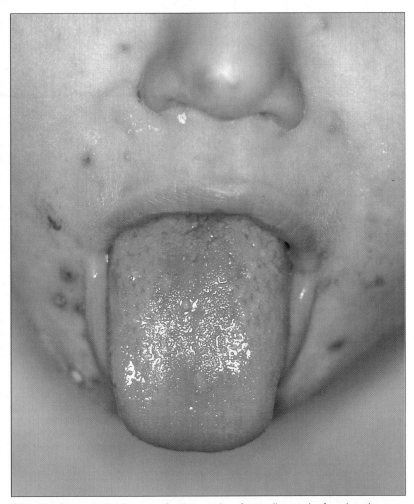

326 Chickenpox in the mouth. The vesicles of varicella may be found on the palate and tongue, and look like minor aphthae. Other causes include viruses like varicella, herpes simplex or microbial infection, Behçet's[58] syndrome, neoplasms, blood disorders, drug reactions and may occur in association with skin disease (lichen planus, pemphigus, and erythema multiforme).

---

[58]Halushi Behçet, Turkish dermatologist, 1889–1948. Über rezidiverende Aphthöse durch ein Virus verursachte Geschwüre am Mund, am Auge und am den Genitalien. *Dermatol. Wschr.*, 1937, **105**: 1152–7. Ulcers of the mouth, genitals and uveitis.

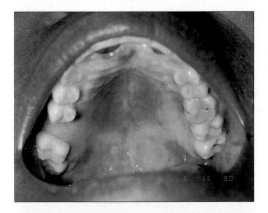

327 Palatal pigmentation. Casual examination of the mouth will miss palatal clues. This black palate with normal pigmented patches should not be confused with Kaposi's sarcoma of the hard palate (*see* **328**).

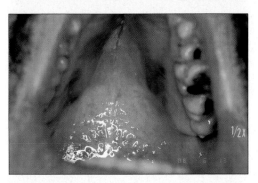

328 Kaposi's sarcoma of the hard palate. Dark red discoloration on the hard palate and a patch of white candidiasis, which must suggest immunosuppression. On a black person dark red rashes look black (*see* **808**, **809**) and the dark red colour of Kaposi's sarcoma[59] on the palate will look black. These are two oral clues to the presence of acquired immune deficiency syndrome (AIDS).The third clue is hairy leukoplakia (*see* **349**). Herpes and stomatitis may also occur in AIDS.

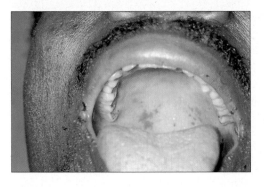

329 Emboli on the hard palate. Petechiae all look the same, but the mouth is an easily missed site. Septicaemia has led to emboli on the palate.

---

[59]Moritz Kaposi-Kohn, Hungarian dermatologist, 1837–1902. Kaposi M. Idiopathisches multiples Pigmensarkom der Haut. *Arch. Derm. Syph.* (Berlin), 1872, **4**: 265–73.

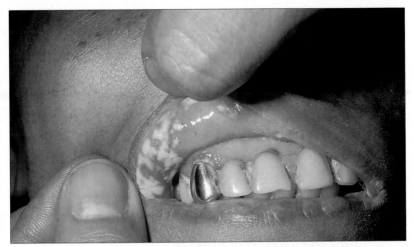

330 *Candida* on the buccal mucosa and gums. Oral *Candida* occurs in immunosuppressed persons. In human acquired immunodeficiency disease (AIDS), infections may appear as the CD4 cell count declines, starting with herpes zoster and then progressing to herpes simplex, tuberculosis, oral candidiasis, Kaposi's sarcoma, *Pneumocystis* pneumonia, atypical mycobacteria and cryptosporidiosis, as the count falls still further.

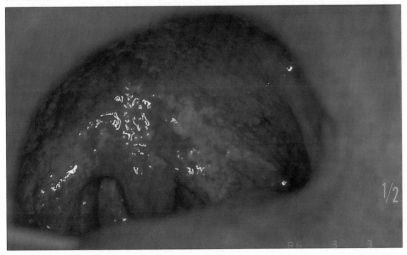

331 *Candida* on the soft palate in asthma. Candidiasis may occur in the immunocompetent – here on the palate in an asthmatic, inhaling corticosteroids, who doesn't rinse the mouth afterwards!

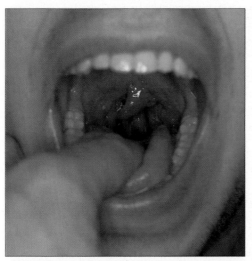

332 Acute tonsillitis. Bacteria or viruses may produce the same inflamed appearance and culture is the only sure discriminating factor unless associated with a scarletina rash on the face.

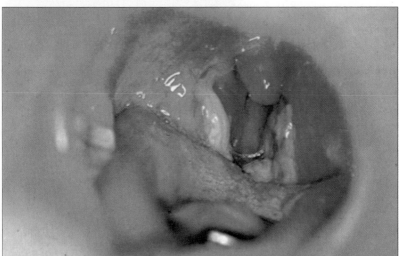

333 Faucial diphtheria—a high index of suspicion. The grey-yellow membrane forms over one tonsil and may spread to involve both, a wrinkled edge bordered with a narrow band of inflammation. Diphtheria may look like any other tonsillitis with a little soreness. From this area the toxin is absorbed to damage distant organs, the heart, peripheral nerves and the kidney. The non-immune (Schick-positive) individual is at risk, yet the immune may show no effects. In developing countries, the disease may be common and in the Russian federation the incidence is increasing.

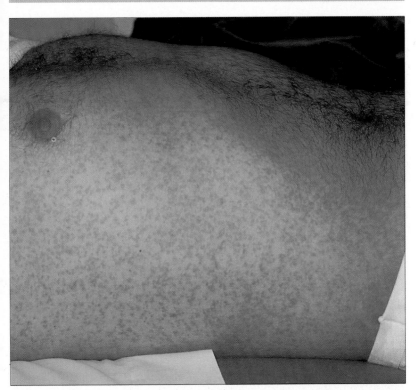

334 Ampicillin in Epstein–Barr[60] virus (EBV) infection. The pharyngitis of mononucleosis due to primary infection with the Epstein–Barr virus, usually affects the more affluent teenager who has been secluded from exposure in childhood. It may be inadvertently treated with ampicillin and show no improvement. The subsequent appearance of the irritating maculopapular rash due to ampicillin hypersensitivity suggests the diagnosis as sensitivity occurs more often with infectious mononucleosis. EBV infection may be associated with Burkitt's lymphoma[61] and other lymphomas in the immunocompromised, some T cell lymphomas, undifferentiated nasopharyngeal carcinoma and oral hairy leukoplakia (see **349**).

---

[60]Epstein MA, British virologist, born 1921. Barr YM, Australian virologist, 20th century.
[61]Dennis Burkitt, British surgeon, 1911–1993. Burkitt DA. Sarcoma involving the jaws in African Children. *Brit. J. Surg.*, 1958, **46**: 218–23.

THE TONGUE

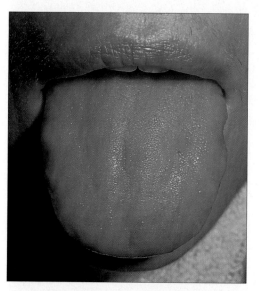

335 A normal tongue.
Pink—haemoglobin 14g/dl—clean, moist and symmetrical, with normal fungiform papillae, which 'taste' the little prominent red papillae sparsely scattered over the anterior part.

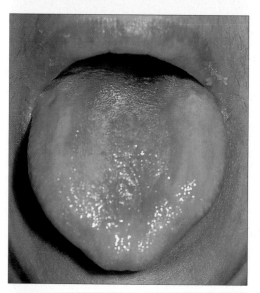

336 A normal tongue.
Many people regard the appearance of the tongue as a barometer of their internal environment. A coated tongue is usually due to substances that have been sucked, eaten or inhaled. Cigarette or pipe smoking gave this characteristic brown colour.

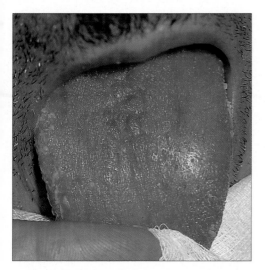

337 A dry dehydrated tongue. Dehydration and mouth breathing may lead to drying of mucus upon it.

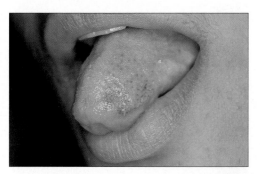

338 The hairy tongue. A black tongue may be due to growth of *Aspergillus niger*.

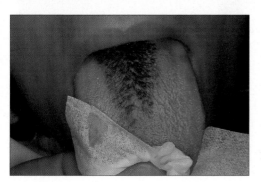

339 A hairier hairy tongue! Growth of *Aspergillus niger* may be prominent and cause anxiety. Reassurance is all that is needed.

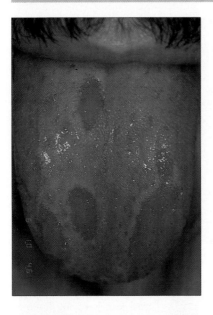

340 The geographic tongue.
Various patterns may appear, looking like an early map in a woodcut atlas, but this benign migratory glossitis is harmless. There is loss of the filiform papillae in patches. The prominent bright red fungiform papillae atrophy if the chorda tympani supplying taste to the anterior two-thirds of the tongue, is damaged.

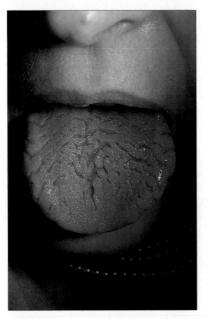

341 The fissured or scrotal tongue. Deep fissures in the normal tongue, but a normal variant.

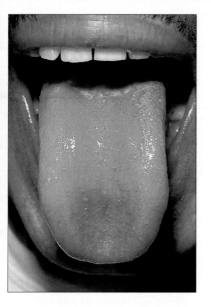

342 Atrophy of the papillae.
Atrophy of the filiform papillae may give this look of atrophic glossitis, which is normal. Compare with **346**, which is certainly abnormal.

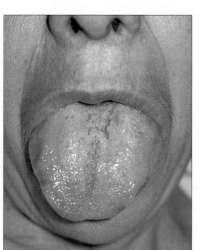

343 The large tongue
(macroglossia). In a small mouth a tongue may seem large. Tooth indentation is seen normally, but prompts thought. Causes include Down's syndrome,[62] cretinism, lymph and haemangiomas in children, and in adults, hypothyroidism, tumours, infiltration with amyloid, and acromegaly—the diagnosis in this patient.

---

[62]John Langdon Haydon Down, English physician, 1828–91. Down JL. Marriages of consanguinity in relation to degeneration of race. *Lond. Hosp. Clin. Lect. Rep.*, 1866, **3**: 224–36. Down JL. Observations on an ethnic classification of idiots. *Lond. Hosp. Clin. Lect. Rep.*, 1866, **3**: 259–62.

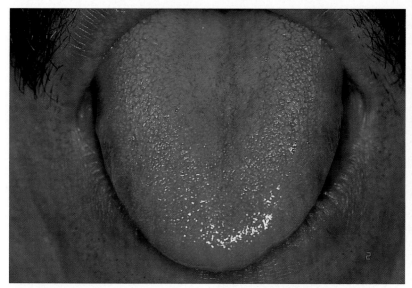

344 Macroglossia. On Christmas eve a television sound engineer complained that he snored, and produced a tape recording of the noises to make his point! He was hoarse and lethargic, with stolid features, and his tongue was big, filling the opening of the mouth—all features of classic **hypothyroidism**.

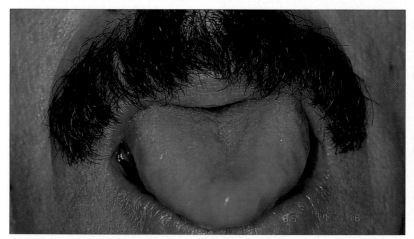

345 Macroglossia—the patient in 344 after treatment. Seven months later, on thyroxine, he no longer snored, was slim and active. His tongue was smaller.

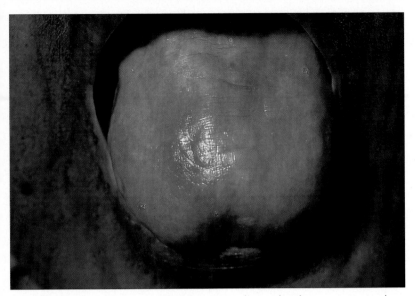

346 Glossitis. A red raw smooth appearance is abnormal and is seen in iron and vitamin B12 deficiency, pellagra, and malnutrition.

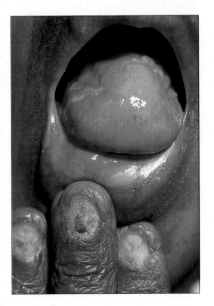

347 Erosive glossitis. A red raw smooth appearance is also seen in association with some skin diseases. The nails have been destroyed and there is severe erosive glossitis and buccal inflammation in **lichen planus.**

165

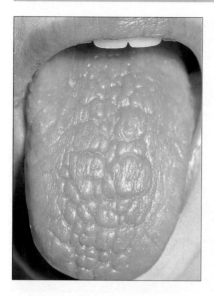

348 The dry tongue. No saliva may result from dehydration due to fluid loss, mouth breathing, or deficient saliva secretion. **The sicca syndrome—**xerostomia—is one component of Sjögren's syndrome (*see* **302**).

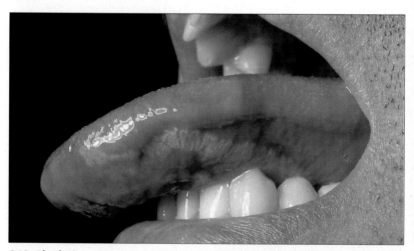

349 The hairy tongue. Latent Ebstein-Barr virus on receptors in the parakeratinised mucosa of the lateral tongue actively replicate in the person immunocompromised with human immunodeficiency virus (HIV). The epithelium becomes shaggy and 'hairy' with vertical white ridges on the lateral margin. This is the appearance of **hairy leukoplakia**. It is not premalignant, but is an important clue to the future development of the acquired immune deficiency syndrome (AIDS).

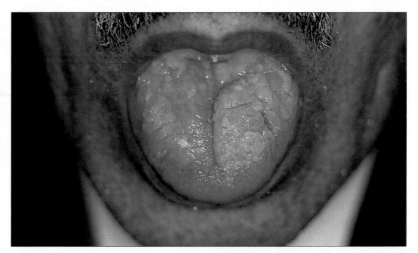

350 A fissured tongue. Superimposed on a fissured tongue are the white plaques of **leukoplakia** (*see* **313**).

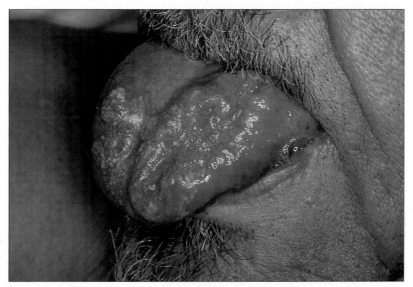

351 Carcinoma of the tongue and leukoplakia. Leukoplakia may develop into a carcinoma. This long-standing pipe and opium smoker presented with a painful tongue ulcer with **leukoplakia**. Biopsy confirmed a diagnosis of **carcinoma**.

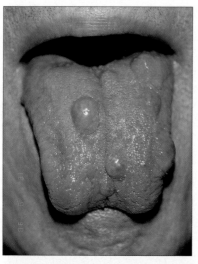

352 Haemangiomas of the tongue. These may be one cause of enlargement, and may be a clue to bleeding elsewhere in the gastrointestinal tract.

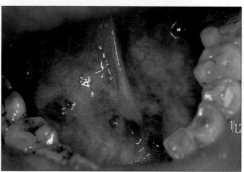

353 Telangiectasia in the floor of the mouth. Macular telangiectatic circumscribed capillary lesions in the mouth may be associated with the common cherry red angiokeratoma of the scrotum—a common finding in the elderly.

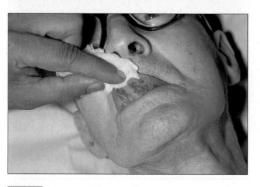

354 Telangiectasia of the mouth and cheek (Osler–Weber–Rendu disease). Telangiectasia of the tongue and cheek are seen in this condition (*see* **46**) and should not be confused with macular telangiectatic circumscribed capillary lesions in the mouth.

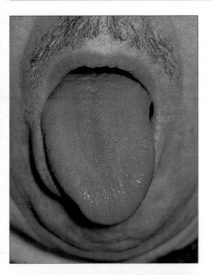

355 The deviated tongue. Deviation will be towards the weaker side secondary to the unopposed action of the normal side. An upper motor neurone (UMN) lesion of the tongue produces mild deviation, and bilateral UMN lesions produce an apparently small spastic tongue. Causes include profound hemiparesis and, if bilateral, pseudobulbar palsy and amyotrophic lateral sclerosis.

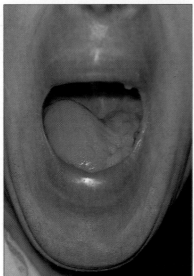

356 The deviated tongue. The wasting of a lower motor neurone lesion of the hypoglossal (12th cranial) nerve produces dramatic wasting when seen in the floor of the mouth.

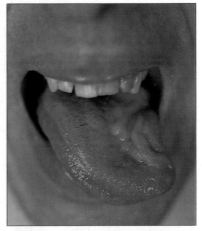

357 Dramatic deviation of the tongue. Deviation towards the paralysed genioglossus. Unilateral lower motor neurone (LMN) lesions of the hypoglossal nerve may be due to trauma, gunshot wounds, brain stem lesions, syringobulbia, tumours or glands at the base of the skull (*see* **209**). Bilateral LMN lesions are a feature of progressive bulbar palsy.

THE HAND

Holding the hand is an active event! An opportunity to assess physical features such as peripheral perfusion and cardiac output while obtaining snippets of the social history by observation and questioning when puzzled. "I see you are left-handed!" when the probability is always right-handed, gives you an opportunity to impress your patient and so gain their confidence.

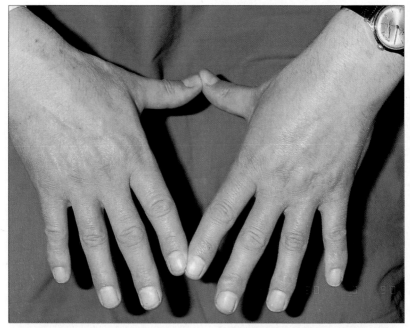

358 The dominant hemisphere—how do you tell? Most people wear their watches on the non-dominant side, so this person may be right-handed, but there is often a confirmatory callus on the medial side of the middle finger where the pen is held (*see* **359**) and here it is on the *left* middle finger. A contradiction because the watch is also on that side! The patient was used to hammering with the right hand and chose to wear the watch on the left.

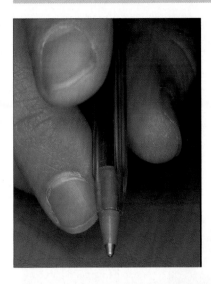

359 Holding a pen. The callus can often be seen over the medial side of the middle finger's terminal phalanx.

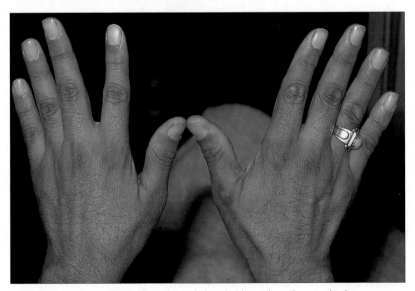

360 Occupation—the tailor. This right-handed bespoke tailor uses his large cutting-out scissors in the right hand and has a callus over the metacarpophalangeal joint from the thumb hole of the scissors' handle and another callus over the ring finger's proximal interphalangeal joint.

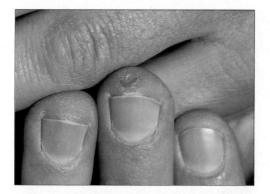

361 Occupation—the guitarist. The left hand exerts pressure on the string of the instrument against the fret to shorten it and change the note. Here is an occupational callus on the tip of the finger.

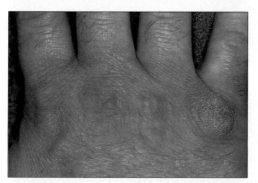

362 Hobbies—the fitness freak. The fitness fanatic who was very heavy found that his wrist hurt if he did 100 press-ups so he supported his body weight on his clenched fists and developed calluses over the knuckles.

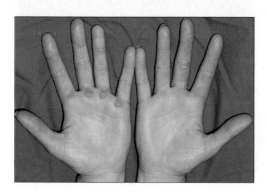

363 Sport—the rower. This elite oarswoman shows the oarsman's palmar thickening. "...The difference in callus is due to the fact that I rowed mainly on bow side—the right hand is used as a hook to pull the oar; the left is used to turn (feather) the oar. There is therefore more friction on the left as more of the left hand is used. The blade goes out to the left. If you look towards the back of the boat where the cox sits, the left-hand side is the bow side." *You get told if you ask!*

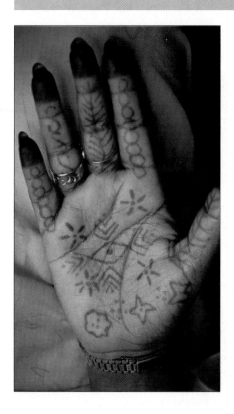

364 Cosmetic colours.

The effect of henna[63], a vegetable dye used to colour the hair and decorate the skin. Patterns of great intricacy may be formed. It was used, to toughen the skin of Arabian Gulf pearl divers, to colour the hair of the elderly, or as an application to the head to relieve headache. On the nails it stains rather than coats, which to the devout Moslem who wishes to wash before prayer, is preferable to nail varnish: henna produces a colouring coat 'permeable' to water and allows cleansing before prayer. The time elapsed since it was applied can be gauged from the amount of undyed nail that has grown out. On the palms, which may be stained when the hair is coloured, the unwary may see pigmented palmar creases and be trapped into invoking an elevated adrenocorticotrophic hormone (ACTH) level as the reason. Modern dyes such as para-phenylenediamine may be mixed with henna to speed up the dyeing process and lead to sensitisation. Henna does not sensitise.

---

[63]The leaves and young shoots of the oriental shrub al-henna (Arabic)—the Egyptian privet. 'Alcanna being greene, will suddenly infect the nailes and other parts with a durable red', Sir Thomas Browne. *Pseud. Epid*, 1646, p.383.

THE MENTALLY DISTRESSED, DISTURBED OR ADDICTED

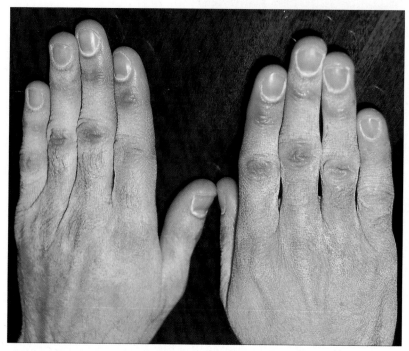

365 The degreased dry hands. This is an effect of excessive cleansing. This is a man with long-standing recurrent abdominal colic and alternating loose stools and constipation (an irritable bowel), but who made no complaint about the hands, which look dry and degreased. As he opened the door, he used a paper tissue to grasp the door knob. Anxiety about germs had led to hourly hand-washing, and rinsing in dilute disinfectant. With the advent of the acquired immune deficiency syndrome (AIDS) his anxiety increased and on re-reading the directions he decided to use undiluted disinfectant. This is an **occult obsessive compulsive neurosis**. In some cases the hands are red and sore, and if the washing extends to cleaning the home, calluses from the broom are seen.[64]

---

[64]Tarsh MJ. Obsessive compulsive neurosis—washing, cleaning and raw red hands. *Br. Med. J.,* 1990, **300**: 888.

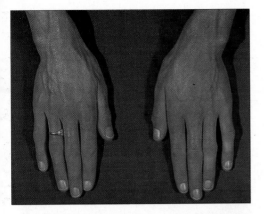

366 Anorexia nervosa.
An increased sensitivity to cold is reflected in the dry, cool and livid skin.

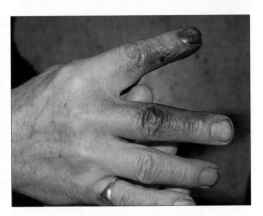

367 The addict—nicotine.
60 cigarettes a day produces obvious staining; even 5–10 a day can be smelt on the fingers.

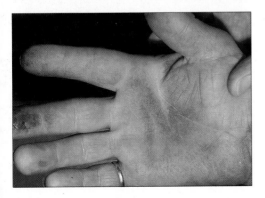

368 The addict—nicotine. Staining of the palm may occur if the cigarette is held with the ignited end between the fingers pointing into the palm and the smoke drifts out of the hollow and stains. A similar palm staining is seen after the use of henna for decoration or applying it to the head to colour the hair.

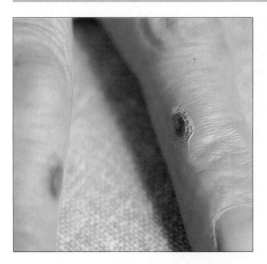

369 The cigarette burn and its significance. This site is typical, where the cigarette is held and burns down, producing a kissing burn on opposed digits. This is a third-degree burn. A blister burn is common, but this full-thickness burn requires anaesthesia! Falling into an alcohol- or drug-induced coma is a common cause.

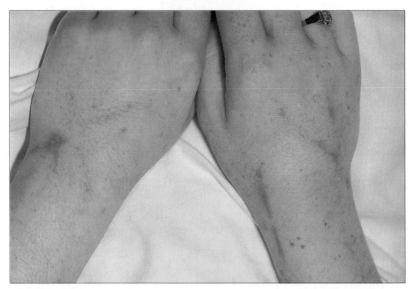

370 The addict—tattoos and drugs. Repeated venepuncture leads to tattooing of the skin over the veins and wrists in a heroin addict. To avoid displaying the stigmata of addiction, other sites are now used. Look for a dimple of tethered skin from repeated puncture of the femoral vein in the groin. Decorative tattoos may be associated with the transfer of infection and hypersensitivity to the pigments.

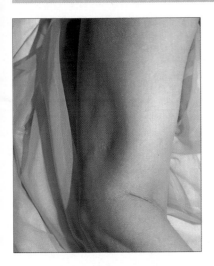

371 The problems of therapy. Fat atrophy (lipoatrophy) at the site of repeated insulin injections in a diabetic may be related to a local allergic reaction to impurities in the insulin. It has become less common with pure insulins. Lipohypertrophy is due to the direct lipogenic action of insulin.

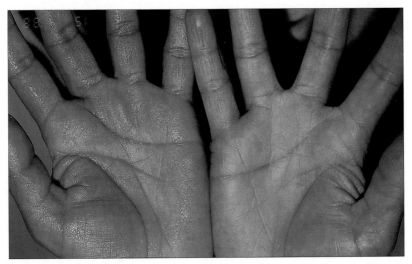

372 The sweaty palm. Hyperhidrosis in a chartered accountant. The normal but hyperhidrotic left hand sweats excessively. As a child he was punished when the chalk on his schoolroom slate was washed away so he could not prove that he had worked out his sums, rather than cheated! Once qualified he had a right sympathectomy to produce a dry hand to greet his clients. Excessive sweating may be due to agents acting on the sweat gland, stimulation of the sympathetic pathway to the gland or stimulation of centres for thermoregulation, gustatory, and mental/emotional sweating.

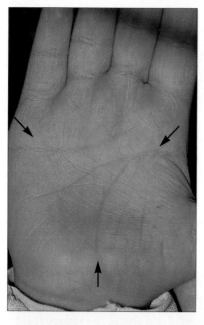

373 The short broad hand.

Changes in dermatoglyphic patterns are related to chromosomal abnormalities. Finger prints are made up of ridges in whorls, loops and arches. At junctional areas the ridges form deltas or tri-radii. The characteristic angle produced by the axial tri-radius in the centre of the palm to the other two demonstrates the broad and short palm in Down's syndrome (trisomy 21) in which the palm is very short and a single transverse crease is present. In Klinefelter's syndrome[65] (47XXY) the ridge count is reduced and in Turner's syndrome[66] (45X) the total ridge count tends to be greatly increased.

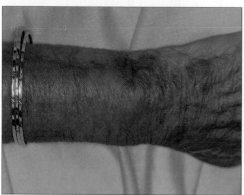

374 Bruises and gold bracelets.

The gold bracelets drop onto the wrist when the arm is moved. Lack of connective tissue support of the blood vessels leads to **senile purpura** and is related to shearing stress. It is more common in association with solar damage and the thin skin that occurs with corticosteroid therapy.

---

[65]Harry Fitch Klinefelter Jr, US physician, born 1912. Klinefelter HF, Reifenstein EC Jr, Albright F. Syndrome characterised by gynaecomastia, aspermatogenesis without A-leydigism, and increased excretion of follicle stimulating hormone. *J. Clin. Endocr.*, 1942, **2**: 615–27.
[66]Henry Hubert Turner, US endocrinologist, 1892–1970. Turner HH. A syndrome of infantilism, congenital webbed neck, and cubitus valgus. *Endocrinology*, 1938, **23**: 566–74.

THE PIGMENTED HAND

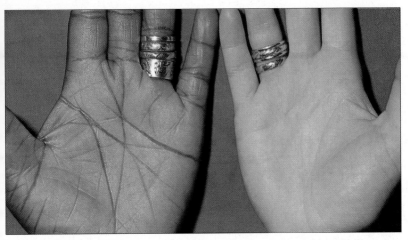

375 An African and a Caucasian palm. Palmar pigmentation is normal in dark-skinned races, but not in Caucasians. On the left an African woman has dark palms and pigmented creases. Indians have pigmented creases too, but Caucasian creases are pink.

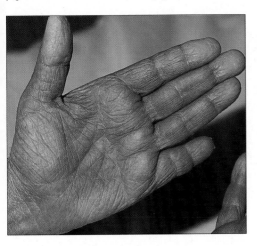

376 Canada–Cronkhite[67] syndrome. Diffuse pigmentation of the volar aspect of the fingers and palms, nail dystrophy and patchy alopecia marks non-hereditary gastrointestinal polyposis. The pigmentation spares the mucous membranes. It may be complicated by diarrhoea and malabsorption.

---

[67]Wilma Jeanne Canada, US radiologist, 20th century; Leonard W. Kronkhite Jr, US physician. 20th century. Generalised gastrointestinal polyposis. An unusual syndrome of polyposis, pigmentation, alopecia and onychotrophia. *N. Eng. J. Med.*, 1955, **252**: 1011–15.

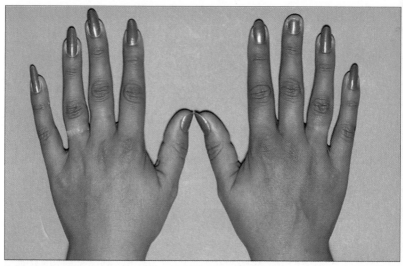

377 A sun-burned girl—1. The hands are tanned. Note the white skin under the finger rings on both ring fingers. The knuckles are dark. She is probably right-handed—on probability and because the index and middle nails are shorter!

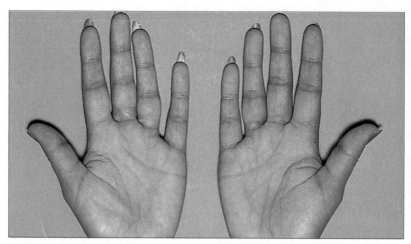

378 A sun-burned girl—2. The palmar creases are darkened. Adrenocortical insufficiency with an excess of adrenocorticotrophic hormone (ACTH) leads to hyperpigmentation.

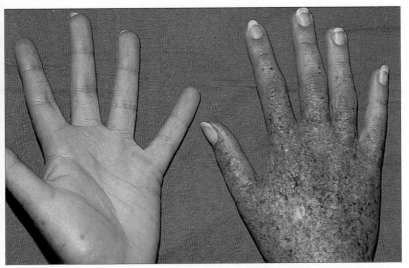

379 Xeroderma pigmentosum. Originally described by Kaposi in 1874[68], an autosomal recessive disease with photosensitivity, premature skin ageing and neoplasia. In contrast to **377**, on this dark skin the dorsum of the hands are pigmented, though the palm is spared. Note the increased freckling and dryness on light exposed surfaces, appearing first on the face and hands. The freckles vary in colour and size and initially fade, later becoming permanent. Gradually telangiectases appear as well as atrophic white spots—malignant tumours may develop early.

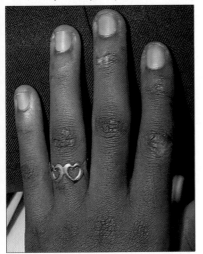

380 Dermatomyositis. Papules over the knuckles (Gottron's papules[69]) and nail bed erythema (*see* **78**). The bluish-red heliotrope rash over the knuckles is black on a dark skin.

[68] Kaposi, M, Hebra, F, On diseases of the skin including the exanthemata. Vol.3 (Tay, W. Trans) *The New Sydenham society*, 1874: 252-8
[69] Heinrich A Gottron, German physician, 1890–1974.

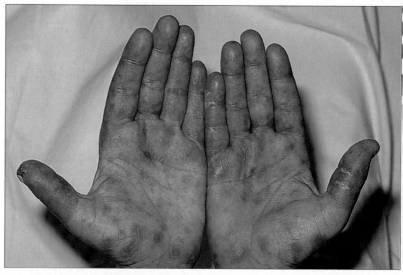

381 Erythema multiforme. Dull red flat maculopapules with a darker centre (iris lesions), which are often seen on the limbs.

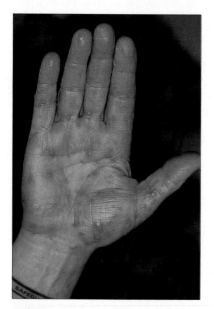

382 Chickenpox. After a hernia operation this 50-year-old developed fever and then a macular papulovesicular rash, with all stages visible in one area. This is chickenpox in a human immunodeficiency virus (HIV)-positive man.

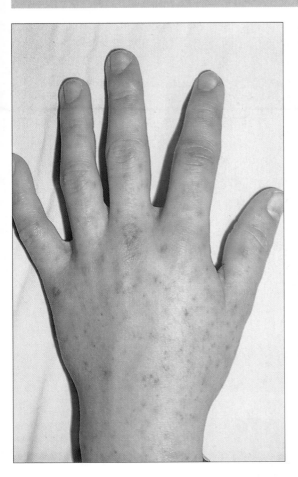

383 Cutaneous vasculitis—Henoch-Schönlein[70] or anaphylactoid purpura. A young girl with abdominal pain, arthralgia, and a palpable purpuric rash with blistering. The arms, legs and ankles were affected by a non-thrombocytopenic purpura with urtication related to immune complex formation to a variety of stimuli. No blood was found in the urine.

---

[70]Eduard Heinrich Henoch, German physician, 1820–1910. Henoch HH. Über den Zusammenhang von Purpura und Intestinalstörungen. *Berlin lin. Wschr.*, 1868, **5**: 517–19. Johann Lukas Schönlein, 1792–1864, *Allgemeine und spezielle Pathologie und Therapie Würzburg*. Etilinger, 1832.

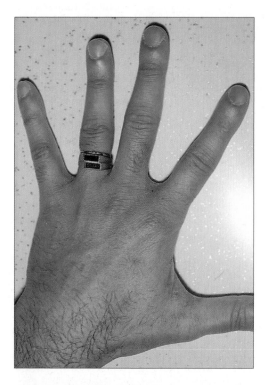

384 Scabies. A barrister with an itchy rash. The finger webs and wrist creases may harbour the scabies mite *Sarcoptes scabiei*, which produces visible burrows on the anterior surface of the wrist and in the finger webs. A vesicle on the thumb is the site of the end of an burrow. She lays her eggs in burrows and dies. The eggs then hatch and the larvae emerge in 3–4 days and make their way to the surface. In 85% of men, mites are carried on the hands and wrists, in 30–40% on the elbows, feet, ankles and genitals. In women, the palms and nipples are favoured.

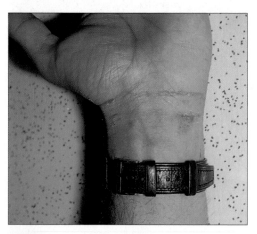

385 Scabies. This is flexural and *not* under the watch strap.

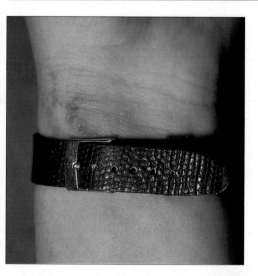

386 Nickel allergy at the watch strap. The scabies shown in **385** should not be confused with **allergic contact dermatitis** immediately adjacent to the nickel buckle. Nickel is a common sensitiser, most commonly in women who react to it in jewellery or fasteners in clothing. It may even be present in detergents.

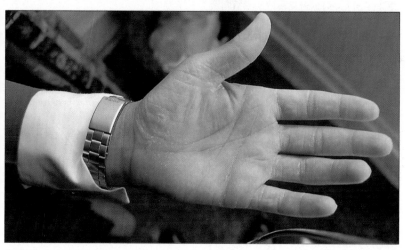

387 Palmar hyperkeratosis. Man cannot function without friction between himself and his environment. Low-intensity friction induces hyperkeratosis leading to calluses, lichenification and pigmentation, whereas high-intensity sudden friction leads to blister formation. Hyperkeratosis may be related to disease or inherited as an autosomal dominant as **diffuse palmar keratoderma** or **tylosis**. It is diffuse, smooth, uniform and may fissure. Acquired keratoderma appearing late in life has been associated with adenocarcinoma of the stomach and bronchial carcinoma.

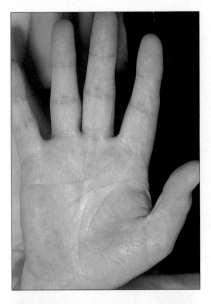

388 Palmar erythema—a pink moist palm. An exaggeration of the palmar redness, palmar erythema may be normal and is seen in pregnancy and in those taking oestrogens. It is also seen in thyrotoxicosis and chronic liver disease. The slight puckering of the palm is mild **Dupuytren's contracture**.[71] The sweating reflects nervousness after an explanation of the technique of liver biopsy.

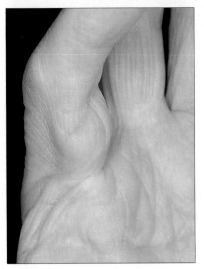

389 Dupuytren's contracture. This is a flexion deformity of the fingers at the proximal interphalangeal joint due to shortening and thickening of the palmar fascia. It affects 2–6% of the population and is more common with increasing age. It may be familial.

---

[71]Baron Guillaume Dupuytren, French surgeon, 1777–1835. Dupuytren G. De la rétraction des doigts par suite d'une affection de l'aponéurose palmaire. Operation chirurgicale, qui convient dans le case. *J. Univ. Hebd. Méd. Chir. Prat.* (Paris), 1833, **5**: 271–3.

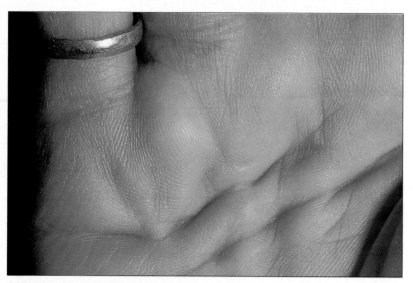

390 Dupuytren's contracture. Nodules may be felt in the palm.

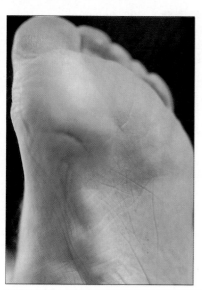

391 Plantar nodules and Dupuytrens's contracture. Nodules may also be felt in the sole of the foot and be associated with knuckle pads and Peyronie's disease.[72] There is an increased frequency among alcoholics (alcoholic cirrhosis) and in diabetics who may also have trigger fingers and stiff hands (**diabetic cheiropathy, *see* 402**).

---

[72]François de la Peyronie, French physician, 1678–1747. Fibrous thickening and curving of the shaft of the penis. De la Peyronie F. Sur quelques obstacles, qui s'opposent a l'éjaculation naturelle de la semance. *Mém. Acad. Chir.* (Paris), 1743, **1**: 425.

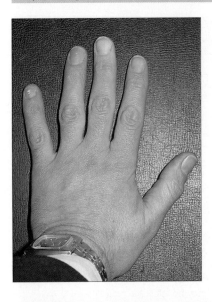

392 Raynaud's syndrome[73]—white. Primary with no underlying disease. Cold and/or emotion produce an intermittent vasospasm of the arterioles in the peripheral limbs. At first the part goes white.

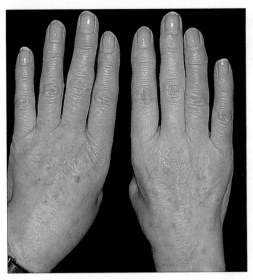

393 Raynaud's syndrome—blue. Primary with no underlying disease. The affected part goes blue after going white.

---

[73]AG Maurice Raynaud, French physician, 1834–1881. *De l'asphyxie locale et la gangrene symetrique des extremities.* Paris, 1862. (Thesis).

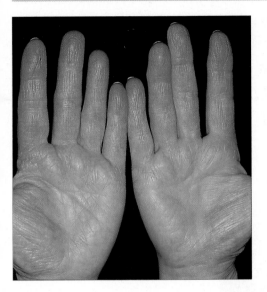

394 Raynaud's syndrome—red. Primary with no underlying disease. The affected part goes red after going blue and then returns to normal.

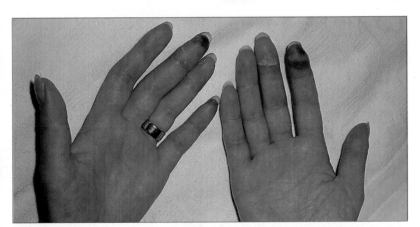

395 Raynaud's phenomenon and gangrene. This severe Raynaud's syndrome progressed to gangrene of the finger. Later the patient developed systemic sclerosis. When associated with an underlying disease, Raynaud's syndrome is called secondary Raynaud's phenomenon or syndrome. The underlying causes to consider include autoimmune diseases (e.g. dermatomyositis, systemic lupus erythematosus, rheumatoid arthritis, and progressive systemic sclerosis), occupational causes (e.g. vibrating tools), nerve compression syndromes at the thoracic outlet and wrist, arterial disease (e.g. thrombo-angiitis obliterans), drugs (e.g. ergot) and gammopathies and cryoglobulinaemias.

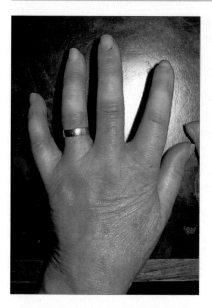

396 Progressive systemic sclerosis (PSS). Raynaud's phenomenon may antedate the appearance of underlying disease by many years. This is secondary Raynaud's phenomenon in systemic sclerosis in which there are the constant changes of PSS (stiff skin and resorption of the terminal phalanx of the index finger) and intermittent vasospastic changes.

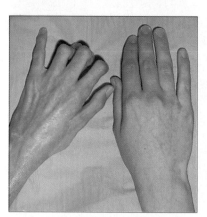

397 Localised morphoea of the hand. Linear morphoea may affect an arm or a leg; if both it is usually ipsilateral. The local sclerosis may extend down to the bone and contractures have developed.

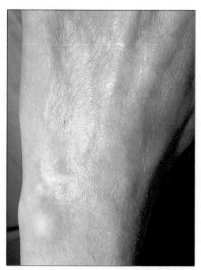

398 The skin texture in localised morphoea of the upper limb. The skin has a waxy shiny surface.

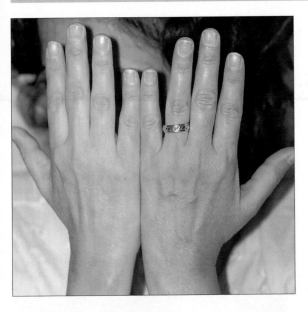

399 Venous obstruction in the arm. The left hand is red compared to the right and there is filling of the veins—both are held above the level of the heart. This woman had secondary deposits in the axilla from a carcinoma of the breast leading to venous obstruction in the arm.

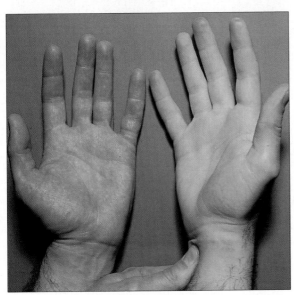

400 Arterial obstruction in the arm. In contrast to **399,** though the affected arm is the same, the colour discrepancy is reversed in arterial obstruction. The hand is again held above the level of the heart and the affected side blanches due to partial arterial embolic obstruction from a subclavian artery aneurysm.

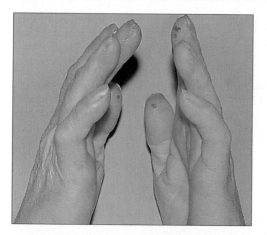

401 Contracture of the little fingers. A common congenital deformity apparent at birth and unrelated to nerve palsy and of no significance, but must be differentiated from other hand postures.

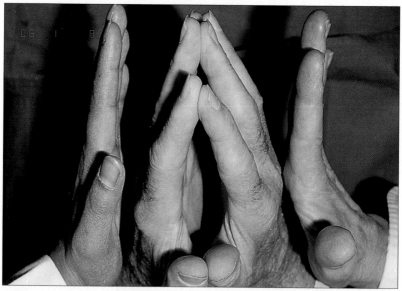

402 The prayer sign. The patient (centre) cannot press the palms of the hands together and oppose the palmar surface of the fingers. The skin has a dry waxy look. On the left is a 22-year-old medical student and on the right a 55-year-old nurse. **Diabetic cheiropathy** in type 1 insulin-dependent diabetes mellitus (IDDM) of long duration is characterised by tight skin, joint restriction and sclerosis of the tendon sheaths—stenosing tenosynovitis. Trigger fingers are common.

WASTING OF THE SMALL MUSCLES OF THE HAND

Important clues can assessed within seconds.

- **Look at the dorsum of the hands.** Is there a local cause or a local clue such as the deformity of rheumatoid arthritis or burns? There is no sensation in syringomyelia.
- **Turn the hands over.** Is the wasting unilateral due to a lesion in the arm or bilateral due to a lesion in the neck or a peripheral neuropathy? Is the wasting symmetrical or is it asymmetrical? Does it affect thenar or hypothenar eminences and is therefore of ulnar or median nerve distribution? Is there a characteristic postural deformity of the median or ulnar nerve or of both nerves?
- **Look at the eyes.** Is there a Horner's syndrome? That places the lesion in the lower chord of the brachial plexus (C8/T1).
- **Look at the face.** If the wasting is thenar, does the patient have acromegaly or myxoedema? Does the patient have features of dystrophia myotonica—frontal balding, cataract and sternomastoid wasting?
- **Look at the feet.** Pes cavus suggests peroneal muscular atrophy (the hands are involved late). Is there unilateral or bilateral foot drop? If so, motor neurone disease or polyneuritis is the cause.

THE SHAPE OF THE HAND

This depends on:
- Wasting.
- Soft tissue overgrowth.
- Bony deformity.
- Posture due to muscle imbalances, which may be fixed or tetanic.
- Nerve innervation—the **median** to the medial aspect and supplying the thenar muscles, and first and second lumbricals; the **ulnar** to the ulnar aspect and supplying the hypothenar muscles, third and fourth lumbricals and all the interossei (T1 segmental supply). Damage to either nerve produces a characteristic posture due to failure of the lumbricals to stabilise the metacarpophalangeal joint, so allowing the extensors to hyperextend at this joint. Thus begins the clawing, which is completed by flexion at the interphalangeal joints as the flexor contracture develops. This leads to clawing of the affected fingers—a good visual clue.

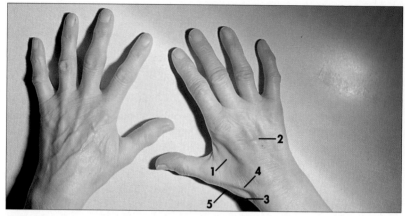

403 The surface anatomy of the hand. The hollow (1) is produced by wasting of **the first dorsal interosseus** muscle; all the interossei are wasted between the metacarpals. This leads to dorsal guttering (2) and is due to either local arthropathy or a peripheral ulnar nerve lesion. Do not describe wasting at **the anatomical snuff box** (3), which is a depression bounded by two tendons—extensor pollicis longus (4) and extensor pollicis brevis (5). The floor is the scaphoid bone. Minor osteophytes on the terminal interphalangeal joints (**Heberden's nodes[74]**) reflect degenerative joint disease. The visible physical sign shown here is **unilateral muscle wasting of the interossei supplied by the ulnar nerve (T1).**

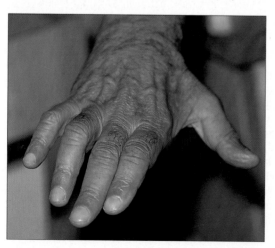

404 A partial claw hand due to an ulnar nerve palsy. There is dorsal guttering, reflecting interosseus wasting and slight extension at the metacarpophalangeal joints of the little and ring fingers as the third and fourth lumbrical muscles are weak.

[74]Sir William Heberden, English physician, 1710–1801. Heberden W. *De Nodis Digitorum*. In: *Commentarii De Morborum Historia Et Curatione*. London, Payne, 1802.

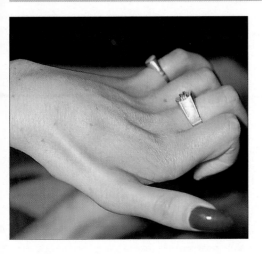

405 The claw hand—main en griffe. A hand gun went off while her friend was cleaning it. Contracture of the paralysed long flexors of the fingers (median and ulnar nerve) with unopposed action of the long extensors without lumbrical balance (median and ulnar nerve) leads to extension at the metacarpophalangeal joint and flexion at the other interphalangeal joints. An ulnar and median nerve palsy due to damage to the lower chord of the brachial plexus producing the full claw hand.

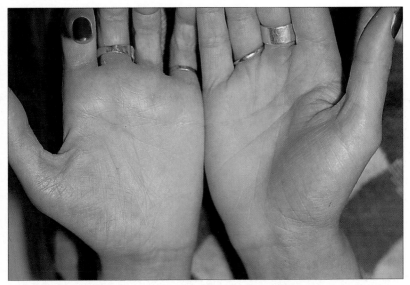

406 Main en griffe. This is the full claw hand shown in **405** demonstrating the flat simian palm with slight finger flexion. The metacarpophalangeal joints are slightly extended and the thumb rotates outward so that it comes to lie in the same plane as the fingers. Compare with the right hand.

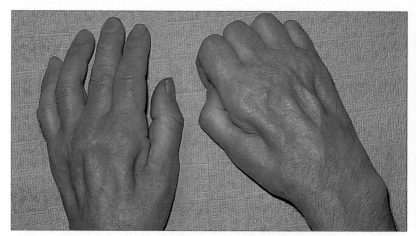

407 Analysing the more complex posture—1. Take one hand at a time. On the left there is the dorsal guttering of interosseus wasting and an ulnar nerve palsy. Look for slight extension at the metacarpophalangeal joints of the little and ring fingers to confirm the **ulnar nerve palsy**. On the right, interosseus wasting produces a picture of ulnar nerve palsy and the hand is contracted with flexed fingers and thumb.

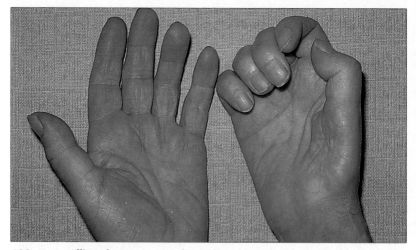

408 Unravelling the more complicated posture—2. Turn the hand over.and note that the left shows slight flexion of the ring and little fingers and some hypothenar flattening, confirming the suspicion of a partial or **ulnar claw hand**. There is thenar and hypothenar wasting of the right hand, suggesting ulnar and median nerve palsies, and as the long extensors are not working, perhaps there is a radial nerve paralysis as well.

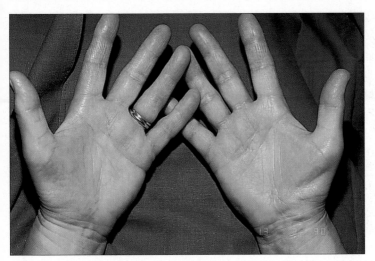

409 A short examination case. This may be considered at either an elementary or advanced level and the solution is in the footnotes. The patient is middle-aged and married and has dry shiny waxy skin—what so far?[75] She has obvious wasting of both thenar eminences affecting abductor pollicis brevis—what so far?[76] So look for what?[77] What else is there—the dry waxy skin, limited extension and the prayer sign is positive. As she attempts to hyperextend her fingers, the tightness of the tissues causes blanching of the fingers. She could be diabetic. Anything else?[78] She has carpal tunnel syndrome, which is half the diagnosis. What is the cause?[79] Can you tie it all together? Have you noticed something on the periphery? Look at the wrists![80]

---

[75] Dry and doesn't sweat so could be elderly or have a peripheral neuropathy. Waxy and dry suggest diabetes mellitus?

[76] Diabetes mellitus and wasting of abductor pollicis brevis on both sides suggest a median nerve lesion on both sides.

[77] The scar of the carpal tunnel release. If there is bilateral carpal tunnel lesion of this severity someone must have realised and operated. There is! So that completes the elementary level diagnosis of carpal tunnel syndrome.

[78] Diabetics with diabetic cheiroarthropathy get stenosing tenosynovitis and if that happens the sheath can be released surgically. Look for a scar, which would be in palm of the hand. There is one on the right at the base of the right middle and ring metacarpophalangeal joints. Another thought confirmed!

[79] Pregnancy?—too old; rheumatoid arthritis or inflammatory joint disease?—no swelling or deformity; acromegaly?—the hands are too slender; myeloma or amyloid infiltration—perhaps, but rare (idiopathic carpal tunnel syndrome in an older age group should always lead to a screen for some form of amyloidosis, particularly myeloma); hypothyroidism?— could be; associated with degenerative joint disease?— could be.

[80] Vitiligo! And what about the association with autoimmune disease? Here is a pointer in favour of hypothyroidism, which was the prime diagnosis. So she has two autoimmune diseases—insulin-dependent diabetes mellitus (and cheiroarthropathy) and hypothyroidism! She also had pernicious anaemia! and a sister with hypothyroidism. A full house—autoimmune disease hunts in packs!

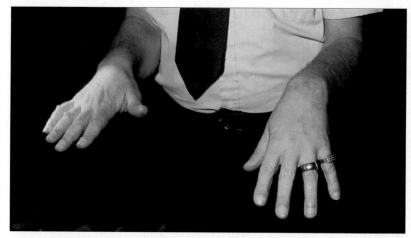

410 Saturday night palsy—1. The pressure of someone's head in bed, crutches or falling into a deep sleep after a night out with the arm over the edge of a chair leads to **radial nerve palsy** due to compression in the spiral groove. This produces a wrist drop.

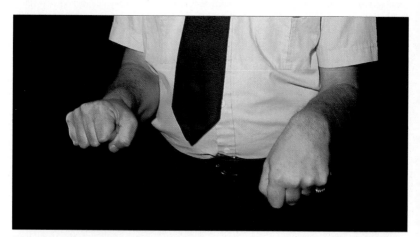

411 Saturday night palsy—2. This also produces an inability to extend the fingers or the wrist when making a fist due to weakness of brachioradialis and the wrist and finger extensors. There is loss of sensation over the base of thumb and first dorsal interosseus. Pure sensory loss and paraesthesiae in this distribution may be due to tight wrist bands—cheiralgia paraesthetica. If radial deviation of the wrist occurs on extension due to weakness of extensor carpi ulnaris, then the purely motor posterior interosseus nerve is at fault.

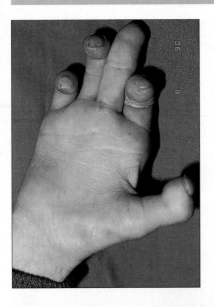

412 A trophic simian hand (*see* **406**). Destruction of the subcuticular pulp and terminal phalanx with extensive trophic changes of the fingers reflects the anaesthetic hand of **tuberculoid leprosy.** Here anaesthesia, dryness and muscle paralysis, aggravated by misuse, have lead to damage from repeated minor trauma to the tips of clawed fingers.

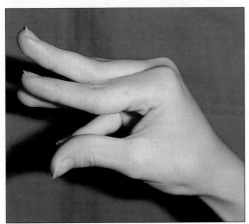

413 Carpal spasm—the accoucheur's hand. Pallor and tetany. This girl felt faint at school, became frightened and began to hyperventilate. Her faintness was related to iron deficiency anaemia. Her fingers are flexed at the metacarpophalangeal joints, the finger tips approximating and the thumb abducted. Carpal spasm may be due to hypocalcaemia,[81] respiratory alkalosis depressing serum ionised calcium, or hypomagnesaemia.

---

[81]A low serum calcium may be due to: absent parathyroid hormone (PTH) in hereditary or acquired hypoparathyroidism; severe magnesium deficiency leading to suppression of PTH secretion; ineffective PTH in chronic renal failure, vitamin D deficiency or defective metabolism; and end-organ insensitivity in pseudohypoparathyroidism; or to flooding of PTH in hyperphosphataemia, tumour lysis and acute renal failure.

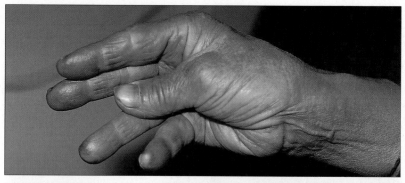

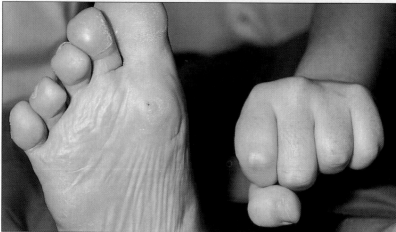

414 (a) Trousseau's sign.[82] A test for latent tetany producing carpal spasm. The dusky appearance and distended veins are due to ischaemia of the forearm from three minutes constriction from a sphygmomanometer cuff. The palmar pigment is henna. **Chvostek's sign** of latent tetany can be elicited by tapping the facial nerve and eliciting a twitch of the face. It is easy to do but non-specific, occurring in 5% of normal people. **(b) The fourth metacarpal and metatarsal are short**. On the sole there is callus from abnormal weight transfer. These are features of **pseudohypoparathyroidism**, but may occur in idiopathic hypoparathyroidism. Somatic abnormalities include short stature, a short neck, short metacarpals and metatarsals. There is end-organ insensitivity to parathyroid hormone. Hypothyroidism may be seen.

---

[82]Armand Trousseau, French physician,1801–67. Noted that a patient being bled for a rheumatic condition developed tetany when the arm bandage was applied. *Clin. Med. Hôtel Dieu* (Paris), 1861, **2**: Baillière Paris.

HANDWRITING

Handwriting is a physical sign and provides clues, for example, the phonetic spelling of a dyslexic person, or a gradual change over time in dopamine deficiency.

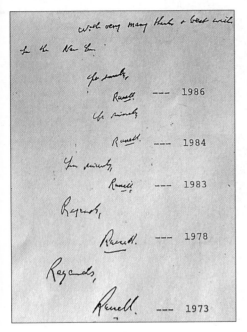

415 A regular Christmas and New Year's card greeting. In 1973 the writing is large. Over the next 13 years the words become smaller and the letters less rounded. Muscle stiffness developed in 1983 and retirement was taken in 1986, by which time the letters become smaller towards the end of the sentence—see the 'e' in 'very' at the start and at the end in 'year'. This is micrographia due to akinesia in **Parkinson's disease**.

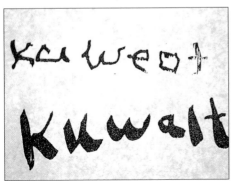

416 Tremor due to mercury poisoning. The mercury rubbed into the scalp as a treatment for hair loss led to poisoning, presenting as ataxia and tremor. She has a fine motor tremor on writing her name and country compared with two years later after therapy, when the tremor had disappeared.

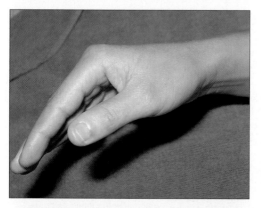

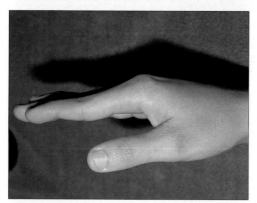

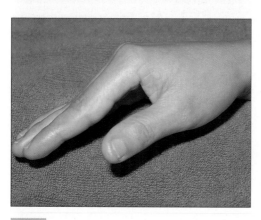

417 The pill rolling tremor. The hand flexes at the metacarpophalangeal joints and extends at the wrist with a frequency of 1–2 cycles/second, with these pictures showing the movement cycle. The tremor of **Parkinson's disease** is first seen at rest and is inhibited by movement, but increased by concentration on a physical or mental task. Anxiety makes it worse. Rest tremor may be due to anxiety, thyrotoxicosis or alcohol, or may be a benign essential tremor. Tremor on movement may be due to essential tremor or cerebellar disease in addition to dopamine deficiency.

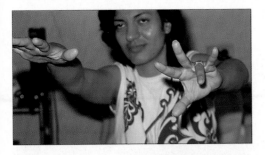

418 Rheumatic or Sydenhams chorea.[83] This produces fidgeting—involuntary variable movements when asked to hold the arm still and outstretched. Note the finger flexion, deviation of the head and pronation of the hand. The movements are unpredictable, brisk, abrupt, and flowing and purposelessly flit about, with twitching and grimacing. It arises several months after a streptococcal infection, affecting children and teenagers, and girls more than boys. It develops insidiously and may be generalised. It resolves over weeks.

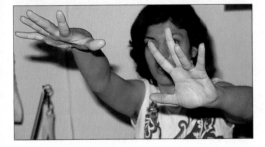

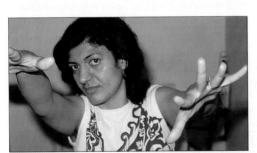

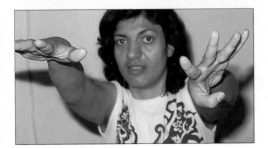

[83]Chorea, Greek for a dance. Chorea Sancti Viti or St Vitus' dance was probably a hysterical manifestation, which spread through Europe in the 15th century (choreamania or dancing madness) and later appended to a disease known by that name. 1686 Sydenham ... *in quae chorea Sancti Viti vulgo appellatur...*

THE SWOLLEN HAND

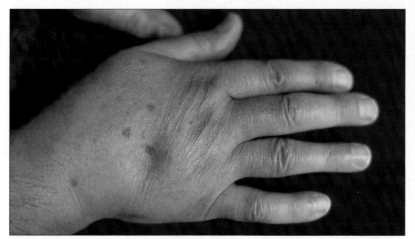

419 'Hair loss, like mown stubble, and puffy hands.' This man had swollen hands and was worried about hair loss on the dorsum. A lack of thyroxine leads to alopecia and a curious broken hair shaft appearance. He had severe **hypothyroidism**, the oedema reflecting increased capillary permeability and disappearing within eight weeks of treatment with thyroxine.

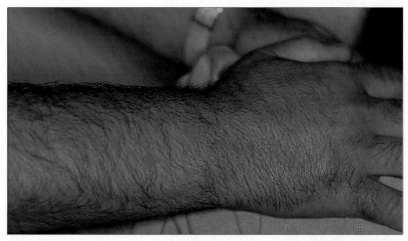

420 Hypothyroidism. The hair regrew after six months of treatment with thyroxine (see figs. **344** and **345**).

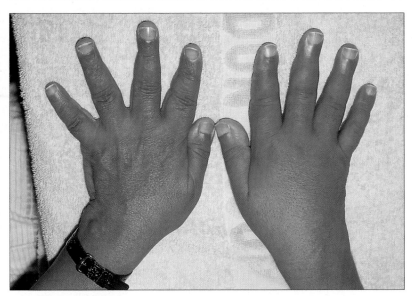

421 The hemiplegic arm. A combination of dependency and a lack of muscular massage of the lymphatics may cause the immobile arm to swell. This also happens if the axillary lymphatics are blocked by metastases or removed surgically.

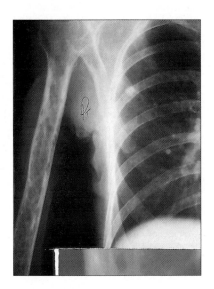

422 Disuse osteoporosis. Disuse may lead to osteoporosis. Here there is bony cystic change affecting the humerus, but not the ribs. The sclerotic margin to the cysts is quite unlike the punched out areas in myeloma. If shown the radiograph of an old febrile person with pneumonia and a high erythrocyte sedimentation rate (ESR), many fall into the trap of an association of ideas (high ESR and bone lesion) with uncritical observation producing the wrong answer. In myeloma the bone lesion is punched out without any edge sclerosis (see **590**).

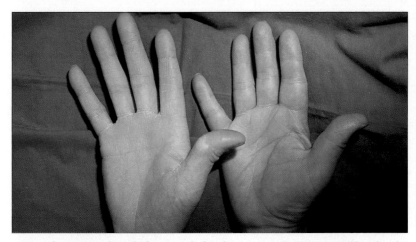

423a The artistic hand—long and slender. A normally proportioned hand (right) and Arachnodactly with long thin fingers and toes in Marfan's syndrome. The patient was 1.88 metres tall and hated the dentist as a child, for his mouth was small and would not open wide. The dentist had difficulties and hurt him.

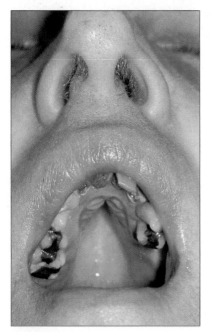

423b Marfan's syndrome—the Gothic or "cathedral roof" palate. At the age of 43 years he developed an abdominal aneurysm and then bilateral popliteal artery aneurysms in the next year. Both his children were also affected, whilst his father died of a ruptured aneurysm at 52. Autosomal dominant inheritance of a mutation of chromosome 15 leads to changes of fibrillin which affect the skeleton, the eye and the cardiovascular system, in particular the elastin containing tissues of the aorta. The relative height (to both unaffected family and the population in general) and the relative length of limbs (to the trunk) is increased. Body habitus, chest deformity (**559**), arched palate (**423b**) and limbs are all clinical markers, but the lens dislocation may only be seen on slit lamp examination. Ascending aortic dilatation may be complicated by aneurysm, aortic valve incompetence or dissection. Spontaneous pneumothorax may occur.

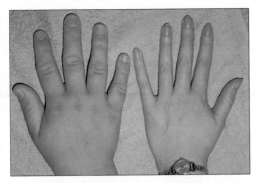

424a A female acromegalic hand and female control. The need for larger gloves in acromegaly is caused by the extra soft tissue which has filled the inter space between the knuckles, fattening this woman's fingers.

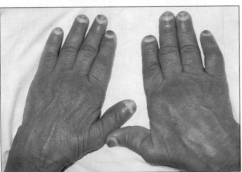

424b The hand increased in size—soft tissue. The coarseness with loss of definition is comparable to the oedematous hand of the hemiplegic. There is henna on the nails, applied at the end of Ramadan, two months earlier!

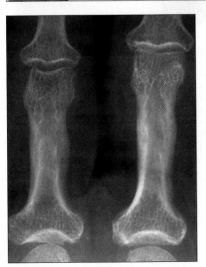

425 Bones in the acromegalic hand. The increase in size is partly related to tufting of the phalanges and an increase in the thickness of the cortex and widening of the joint space.

VITAMIN D DEFICIENCY

The groups most at risk of vitamin D deficiency—Asian immigrants and the elderly—are those with a low intake of vitamin D and low 25-hydroxy vitamin D levels. The vitamin D deficiency may be due to:

- deficient synthesis in the skin due to a lack of sunlight, which is aggravated by pigmentation and affected by malabsorption induced by the presence of a high extraction flour in the diet and *particularly* by the extent to which the diet is vegetarian.
- metabolic interference with 25-hydroxylation in chronic liver disease and increased breakdown of vitamin D when on anticonvulsants.
- renal disease that interferes with 1-alpha hydroxylation in the kidney.[84]

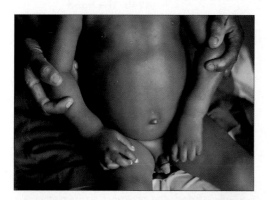

426 Swollen wrists. This child walks with difficulty. The wrists show bilateral swelling of the lower radial epiphysis.

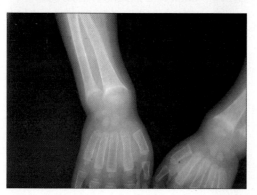

427 Swollen wrists— radiograph. The clinically expanded junction is due to an increase in uncalcified osteoid at the widened and cupped epiphysis of the lower end of the radius. This is **vitamin D deficiency rickets** affecting the growing skeleton.

---

[84]Henderson JB *et al.* Asian osteomalacia is determined by dietary factors when exposure to u/v radiation is restricted. A risk factor model. *Quart. J. Med.*, 1990, **76** (261): 923–33.

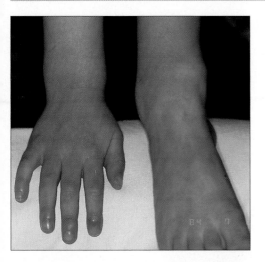

428 Swollen wrist and ankle. This young girl was an immigrant from South East Asia and living in a town in the north of England. The ankle and wrist are widened immediately above the joint line and a second prominence is seen above the wrist crease and the malleoli (vitamin D deficient rickets).

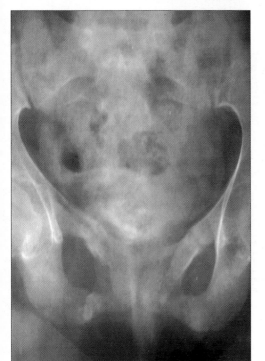

429 Vitamin D deficiency. This elderly lady has pain on walking, particularly on climbing stairs. Osteomalacia of the mature skeleton leads to limb girdle muscle weakness and Looser's zones, which are seen here in the pubic rami as a ribbon fracture (an area of demineralisation) and often along the medial edge of the femur.

OTHER BUMPS ON THE HAND

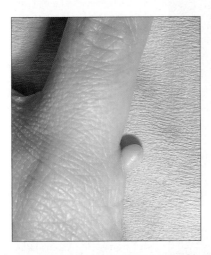

430 The accessory digit. Twelve-digit woman—a curious anomaly ranging from rudimentary appendages to complete six finger hands.

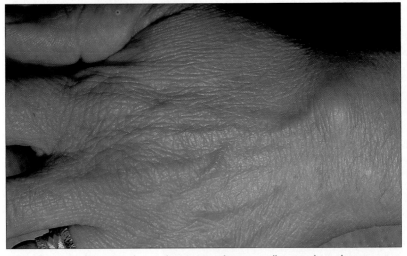

431 The ganglion. People may be anxious about a swelling overlying the wrist joint that may come and go or be reduced by firm pressure. This is a cyst of the synovial membrane and is traditionally cured by hitting it with the family bible. It is seen on the anterior aspect of the wrist and in rheumatoid arthritis may be ballotted from the palm to the flexor tendons (**a compound palmar ganglion**).

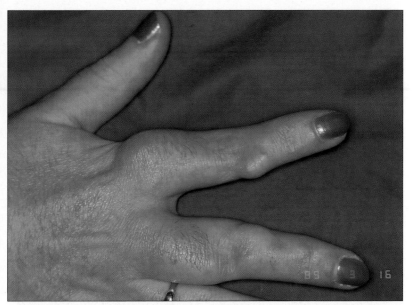

432 Ollier's disease (enchondromatosis). The presence of haemangiomas, and lumps produced by expanded cartridge islands[85] must be differentiated from the picture produced by asymmetrical growth due to cartilage islands distorting the growth plate.[86] In the terminal phalanx they may look like a solitary bone cyst.

---

[85]Maffucci's syndrome. Angelo Maffucci, Italian pathologist, 1845–1903. Di un caso encondroma et angioma multiple. *Mov. Med. Chir.*, 1881, **3**: 399.

[86]Ollier's syndrome. Louis Xavier Edouard Leopold Ollier, French surgeon, 1830–1900. Ollier LXEL. De la dyschondroplasie. *Bull. Soc. Chir. Lyon*, 1899–1900, **3**: 22–7.

OSTEOARTHRITIS IN THE HAND

In the hand, osteoarthritis affects the terminal interphalangeal joints, the proximal interphalangeal joints, the carpometacarpal joint of the thumb, and the metacarpophalangeal joints in order of frequency.

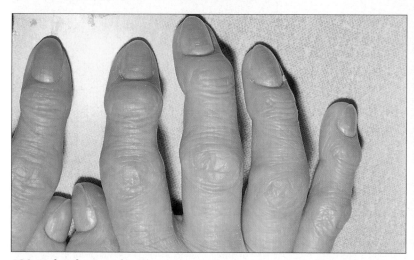

433 Heberden's nodes. These are osteophytes on the dorsum of the terminal interphalangeal joints and called Bouchard's nodes[87] on the proximal interphalangeal joints. Differentiate from rheumatic nodules (*see* **448**), tophi (*see* **463**) and synovial cysts (*see* **435**).

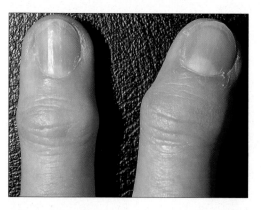

434 Heberden's nodes. Classical nodes in a male. Osteoarthritis affects the hand with a sex incidence of males to females of 4:1. At the base of the thumb this figure is 6:4, whilst at the wrist it is 1:4. The deviation of the joint is due to asymmetrical loss of cartilage.

[87]Charles Jacques Bouchard, French physician, 1796–1881.

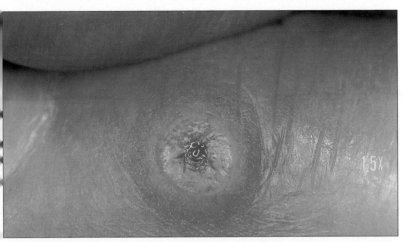

435 A mucous cyst over the terminal interphalangeal joint. These cysts may form around the early osteoarthritic joint and be accompanied by pain, which is relieved when the glairy synovial fluid is released on rupture.

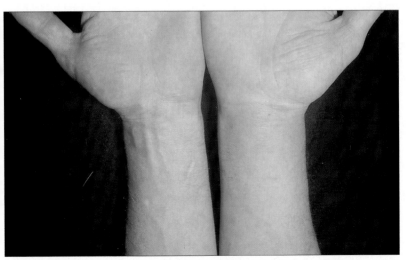

436 Palindromic—'running backward'—rheumatism. This 40-year-old man had recurrent acute attacks of pain in one or both wrists and hands, reverting to normal after one or two days. He has no associated systemic or blood abnormality. The differential diagnosis includes rheumatoid arthritis, gout, pseudogout and a collagen disease. Rheumatoid arthritis may develop later.

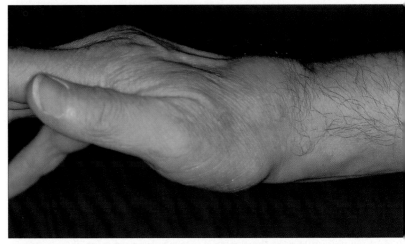

437 Synovial thickening at the wrist—rheumatoid arthritis. The swollen wrist and thickened synovium feel 'boggy' and there is a characteristic deformity, which is usually greater on the ulnar side. The tenosynovitis may lead to later tendon rupture.

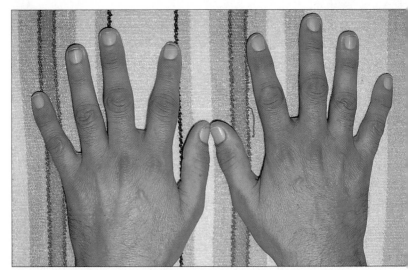

438 Polyarthritis of the hands. The distribution of early rheumatoid arthritis affecting the proximal interphalangeal and metacarpophalangeal joints. The index finger has a characteristic fusiform shape.

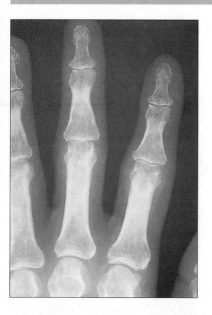

439 Fusiform or spindled fingers.
Radiologically soft tissue swelling is
present and periarticular rarefaction of
bone has occurred.

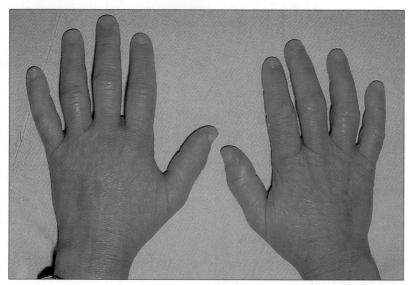

440 Polyarthritis of the fingers—systemic lupus erythematosus. Swelling of
all the interphalangeal joints with less marked spindling.

CLASSIC HAND DEFORMITIES OF RHEUMATOID ARTHRITIS

Joint disruption and collateral ligament instability leads to typical deformities.

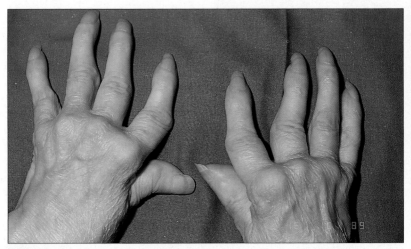

441 Rheumatoid ulnar deviation and metacarpophalangeal joint subluxation. Metacarpophalangeal joint involvement leads to volar displacement with subluxation.

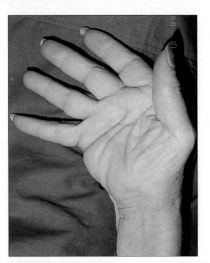

442 Ulnar deviation of the fingers. Metacarpophalangeal joint involvement also leads to ulnar drift as the power of the grip pulls the tendons towards the ulnar. The linkage of the extensor tendons means that the pull on the fifth extensor tendon will be transmitted to all the other fingers and pull them in the same direction.

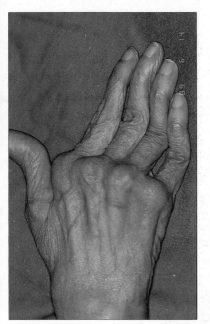

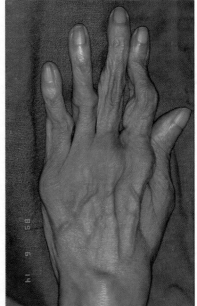

**443 Ulnar deviation guttering—
swan neck fingers.** Ulnar drift is
associated with wasting of the interossei
from pain and disuse, whilst there is a
swan neck deformity of the fingers (*see*
445).

444 The boutonnière finger.[88] Lack
of support from collateral ligaments leads
to proximal interphalangeal joint
instability. This is seen in the index
finger— the central slip weakens and the
lateral bands slip down and become
flexors at the proximal interphalangeal
joint with extension concentrated at the
terminal interphalangeal joint. The middle,
ring and little finger show swan neck
deformity.

---

[88]Buttonhole mechanism. If inflammation leads to weakness of the central slip of the extensor insertion into
the base of the middle phalanx, the proximal interphalangeal joint may protrude between the lateral
extensions of the extensor tendons like a button through its hole, with the extensors acting as flexors
across the joint.

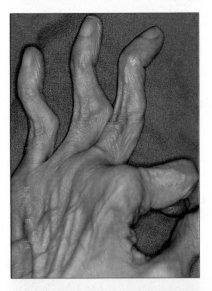

445 The swan neck finger.[89] This is the reverse of the boutonnière deformity with the lateral bands seen subluxing upwards. Once fixed, flexion may become impossible.

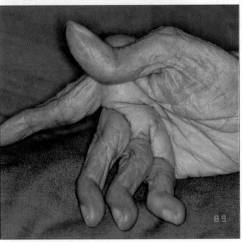

446 Z deformity of thumb.. Deformity of the thumb in rheumatoid arthritis leads to hyperextension of the interphalangeal joint in the same way as **443** producing hitchhiker's thumb.

---

[89]Hyperextension at the proximal interphalangeal joint with flexion at the terminal interphalangeal joint. Forward subluxation of the metacarpophalangeal joint results in tightening of the intrinsic muscle, which in turn causes the metacarpophalangeal joint to flex as finger extension occurs. But if there is destruction of the volar plate of the proximal interphalangeal joint, the hyperextension occurs here. The distal interphalangeal joint is flexed because the pull of the extended profundus tendon exceeds that of the long extensor tendon, two lateral slips of which can be seen bowstrung across the proximal interphalangeal joints.

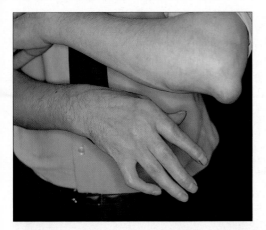

447 Olecranon bursitis, nodules and a rheumatoid hand. This patient is a heavy cigarette smoker with seropositive rheumatoid arthritis. Features include an olecranon bursitis, rheumatoid nodules along the subcutaneous ulna border, synovial thickening at the wrist, ulnar drift of the fingers and early subluxation of the fifth finger. The rheumatoid synovitis of the bursa may become a portal for systemic infection. Contrast this with **460**.

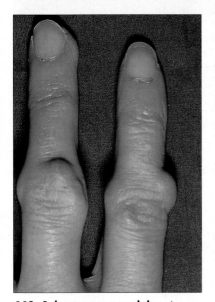

448 Subcutaneous nodules. A diagnostic marker of rheumatoid arthritis affecting 30% of patients. They are usually seen over bony pressure points and prominences. They may be present over the fingers, ischial tuberosities (*see* **648**) or occiput. They may ulcerate.

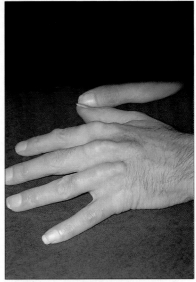

449 Tendon nodules. The subcutaneous nodules of rheumatoid arthritis should not be muddled with tendon nodules due to **xanthomas** in hyperlipidaemias.

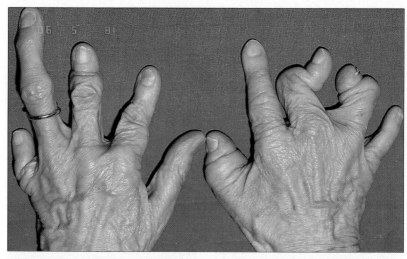

450 Psoriatic arthritis (arthritis mutilans). A nun with 11 pairs of pristine custom-made surgical shoes, who thought it thrifty not to wear them out of doors. Long-standing seronegative arthritis and nail changes, but no skin rash. Onycholysis or separation of the nail from the bed is seen at the nail edge and as oil drop patches of the index, both ring fingers and thumb.

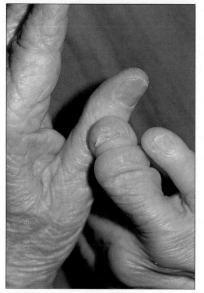

451 Lorgnette or telescope finger and salmon patch on nail. The asymmetrical joint destruction leads to telescoping of the digits.

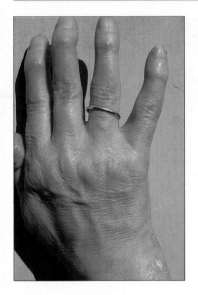

452 Terminal digital swelling and psoriasis. Psoriatic arthritis is more often seen as the characteristic terminal interphalangeal swelling with coexisting nail changes, pitting and onycholysis, and a plaque of psoriasis at the wrist. Heberden's nodes and psoriasis may coexist and lead to confusion. Other manifestations may include oligoarthritis, sacroiliitis and a single swollen digit.

THE SWOLLEN DIGIT

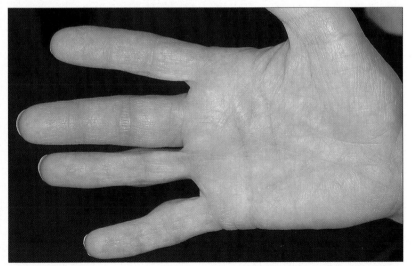

453 Sausage finger. The sausage shape arises from swelling of the tendon sheaths and all the joints of the finger or toe. A similar change may be found in reactive arthritis.

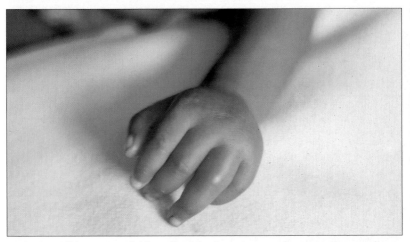

454 Dactylitis—acute sickle cell crisis. Bone marrow infarction in the carpals, tarsals or phalanges leads to severe pain and oedema in this haemoglobinopathy—the hand–foot syndrome.

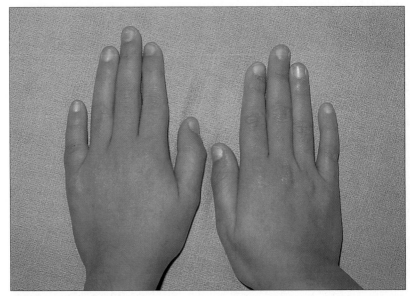

455 Dactylitis residua. A short left little finger. In adult life the residual deformity can lead to the suspicion of an abnormal haemoglobin. Compare with **778**.

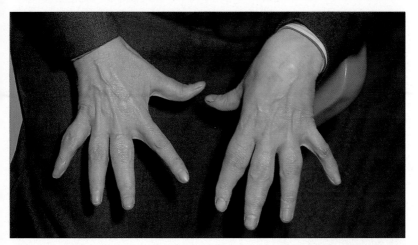

456 Sarcoid bone cysts in the fingers. This woman with a dull blue-red plaque on her face and markedly swollen but painless fingers has bone cysts and lupus pernio due to sarcoidosis.

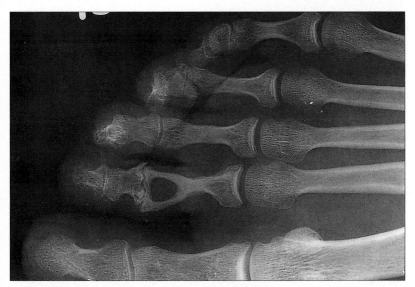

457 Radiograph of bone cysts in the proximal phalanx of the toe. A single bone cyst in a digit. While an enchondroma can mimic a bone cyst in the digit, the presence of haemangiomas confirms Ollier's disease.

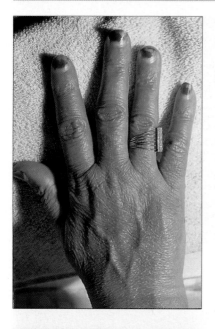

458 The swollen hand in hyperparathyroidism. This woman presented with epigastric pain and ascribed the swelling of the ulnar side of her hand to trauma because she had shut it in a car door one month earlier. She had a duodenal ulcer.

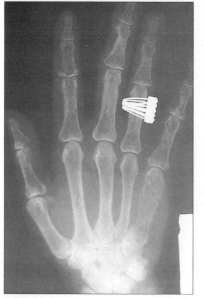

459 Radiograph of the hand shown in 458. There was chondrocalcinosis of the knees and, in the hand, osteoporosis, bone cysts in the fifth metacarpal joint and subperiosteal erosions in the fifth and index fingers. A parathyroid adenoma was removed.

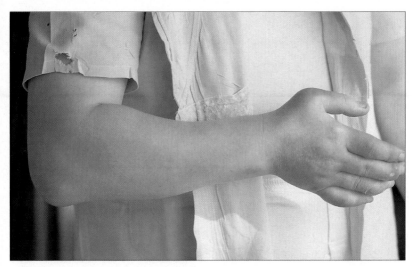

460 Gout of the hand—tophi on the elbow. The tophus on the elbow mimics an olecranon bursa, the fingers are sausage shaped, and the squaring of the base of the thumb is due to osteoarthritis, but tophi are seen on the fingers (*see* **463**).

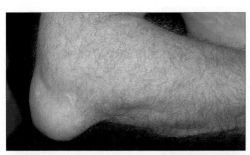

461 The olecranon bursa. A South African retired rugby player was told by his surgical friend that his olecranon bursa was best removed surgically. He demurred, and his wife, a nurse, agreed.

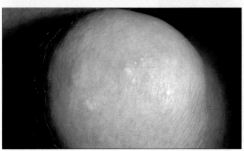

462 Close-up of the elbow shown in 461. Careful examination of the skin shows the urate of this tophus showing through the skin. Olecranon bursae may be traumatic or due to sepsis (and can progress from the former to the latter), related to gout, or due to a rheumatoid synovitis.

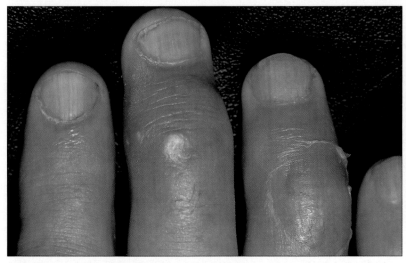

463 Gouty tophi of the fingers. Warmth, redness, pain, swelling, and a discharge with postinflammatory desquamation is easily confused with infection.

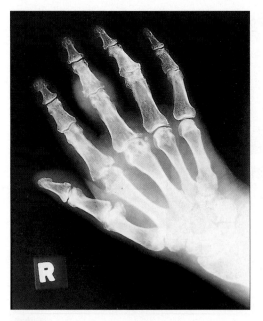

464 Radiograph of a hand with tophaceous gout. This shows the radiolucent tophaceous soft tissue swelling and punched out erosions with no juxta-articular osteoporosis, so confirming tophaceous gout.

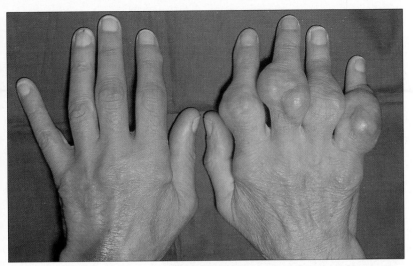

465 Tophi on the hands. Unilateral swellings lie over the proximal phalanges. The yellow–ivory colour of the urate shows through the skin over the fifth finger tophus.

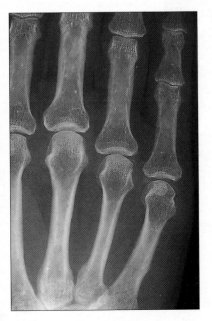

466 Chondrocalcinosis in the hand. The calcification seen in the joint space of the fifth metacarpophalangeal joint may be a clue to the presence of gout, pseudogout, hyperparathyroidism, Wilson's disease, haemochromatosis or degenerative joint disease (*see* **21**).

THE NAIL

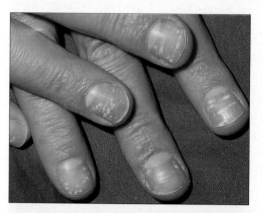

467 Punctate leukonychia. White marks on the nail are common and may be punctate, striate, and even complete. They may be related to trauma, but usually no cause is found. They need to be distinguished from the whiteness due to fungal infection and that associated with hypoalbuminaemia.

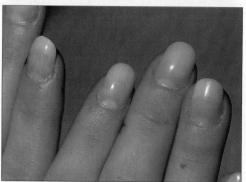

468 White nails. The unworldly male must not fall into the trap of diagnosing white nails when in fact these nails are false, disguising the bitten nails.

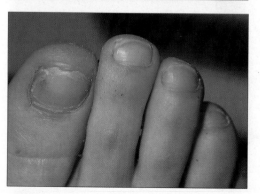

469 Her toes. The girl whose nails are shown in **468** compensated by tearing off her toe nails!

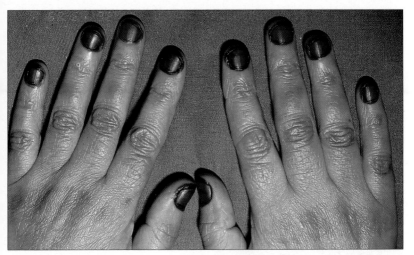

470 Henna on the nails. Henna, freshly applied, stains the skin and nails. The colour will disappear from the skin quickly, but that on the nail will remain until the nail grows out (*see* **364**).

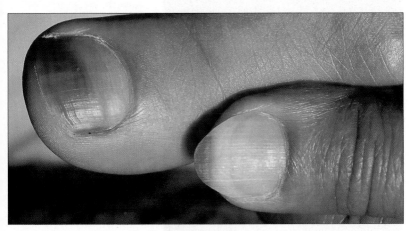

471 Nail growth as a clock—Quitter's nail. The finger nails grow at a rate of 1–2 mm a week, the toes more slowly. The stain was applied to both on the same day. An identical appearance *after* stopping smoking (nicotine staining) may be seen in the successfully reformed cigarette smoker (Quitter's nail[90]).

[90]Verghese A. Images in clinical medicine—Quitter's nail. *N. Eng. J. Med.*, 1994, **330**(14): 974.

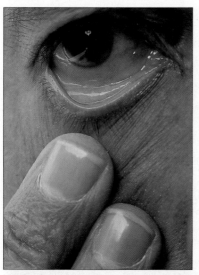

472 The shiny nail due to obstructive jaundice. This is the sign of the chronic scratcher (the chronic pruritic). When you itch, the nail tip is used and after about four weeks of scratching the distal third of the nail becomes buffed like a mirror—the roof line of the houses outside is reflected in his eye *and* in his nail tip—whereas the proximal end remains matt. The diagnosis may range from senile pruritus to scabies and includes malignancy, cholestasis, diabetes mellitus and neurodermatitis. So a combination of chronic pruritus and jaundice indicates cholestasis.

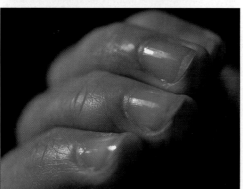

473 Shiny nail—clear varnish. In contrast to **472**, the manicured nail with clear nail varnish has a gloss extending to and slightly onto the cuticle!

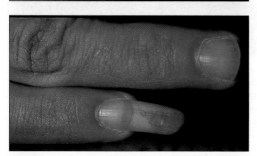

474 An auricular digit. For cleaning the ears.

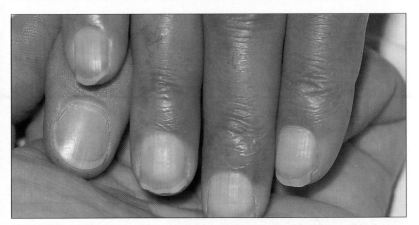

475 White nails. On the left is a normal nail. The opacity of the white nail bed obscures the lunula. There is a band of normal pink distally.

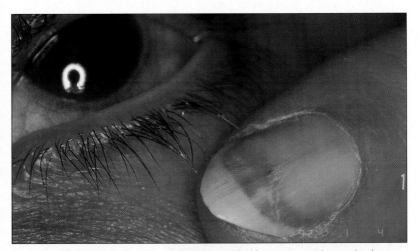

476 The half and half nail—a diabetic with glaucoma.. When wider than that shown in **475**, the band of distal pink gives the appearance of the half and half nail or **Terry's nails**.[91] The association with cirrhosis is tenuous. This change may be found in a quarter of hospital inpatients and in cirrhosis, congestive cardiac failure and diabetes mellitus, as well as in the elderly. The band is due to distal telangiectasia.[92]

---

[91] Terry R. White nails in hepatic cirrhosis. *Lancet*, 1954, **i**: 757–9.

[92] Holzberg M, Walker HK. Terry's nails. Revised definition and new correlations. *Lancet*, 1984, **i**; 896–9.

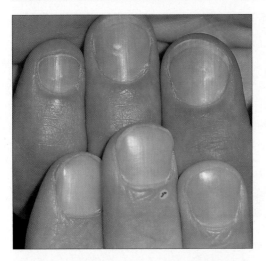

477 Pallor of the nail bed. Compare the normal nail bed (with punctate leukonychia) and the pale capillary bed of the severely anaemic patient (Hb 9g/dl—*see* **10, 11** showing the buccal mucosa of this man).

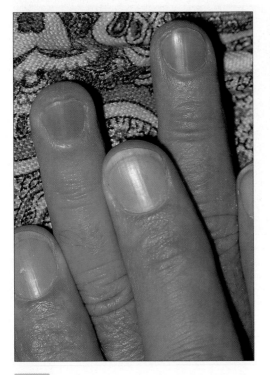

478 Grey nails. Change in nail colour may be due to stain or varnish, or reflect pigmentation due to argyria and melanin. This man had disseminated melanomatosis and developed a grey tint.

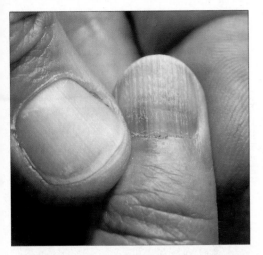

479 Chromonychia and drugs. This woman underwent chemotherapy for lymphoma and her nails became coloured during treatment. Such a colour change is common during cytotoxic therapy. As a result of therapy there is a depression due to growth arrest of the nail—ridging and beading cease at the junction.

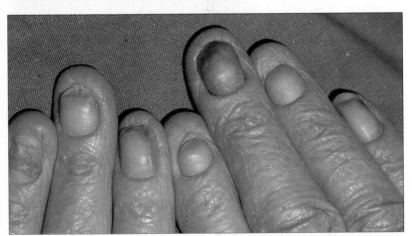

480 The yellow nail syndrome.[93] This 70-year-old woman has recurrent chest infections and oedema of the feet. These yellow–green nails are thickened and curved excessively from side to side, have no cuticle, and grow slowly. Onycholysis may spread to the nail plate and the nail is shed, but may regrow. There is often limb oedema and associated chronic bronchitis, pleural effusions and bronchiectasis.[94] Complete spontaneous recovery has been seen.

[93]Samman PD, White WF. The yellow nail syndrome. *Brit. J. Derm.*, 1964, **76**: 53.
[94]Emerson P. Yellow nails, lymphoedema and pleural effusions. *Thorax*, 1966, **21**: 247.

The nail bed

The nail bed may reflect vasculitis in rheumatoid arthritis (*see* **485**) and infarcts in progressive systemic sclerosis (*see* **486**) as well as dilated capillary loops (*see* **502**) in other collagen diseases, such as systemic lupus erythematosus and dermatomyositis.[95]

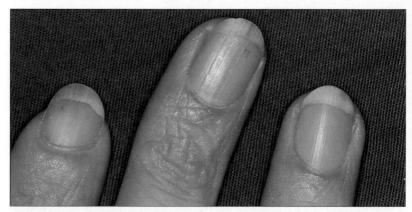

481 Splinter haemorrhages. These longitudinal haemorrhages under the nail are easily overlooked until you look closer.

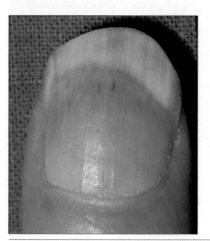

482 Splinter haemorrhages in close-up. They may be few or many and occur in 26–56% of normal people as a result of trauma. They are more common on the right hand and more frequent in manual workers and in psoriasis. They decline in frequency with the duration of a long inpatient stay. Splinter haemorrhages may be seen in bacterial endocarditis, but are often absent, and in those with indwelling arterial lines.[96]

---

[95]Samitz MH. Cuticular changes in dermatomyositis. *Arch. Dermatol.*, 1974, **11**: 866.
[96]J.B. Young *et al.* Splinter haemorrhages: fact and fiction. *J. Roy. Coll. Phys. Lond.*, 1988, **22**: 4, 240.

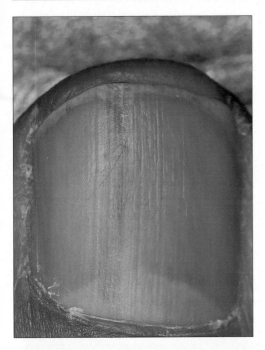

483 Linear or junctional nail matrix naevus.
Pigmented bands are common in dark-skinned people.

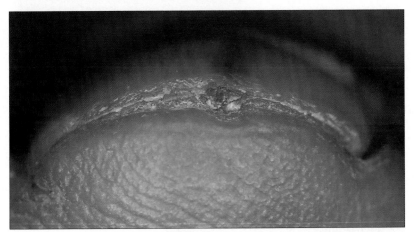

484 End-on view of a linear naevus of the nail. In a white-skinned person a band may be produced by a junctional nail matrix naevus, which has a potential for malignancy, or a melanoma. A linear naevus may darken in adrenocortical insufficiency.

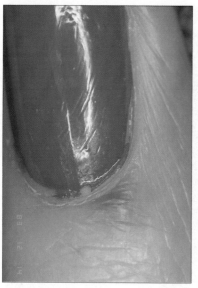

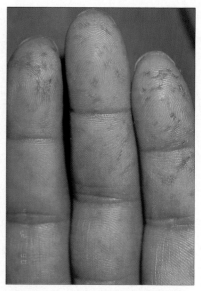

485 Nail varnish and vasculitis.
An early vasculitic lesion at the nail base in rheumatoid arthritis. These may progress through a cycle to infarction.

486 Finger pulp infarcts. Full-blown pulp infarcts in systemic sclerosis. The infarcts are seen in different stages, some as red areas, some dark and depressed, and some dry or sloughed out (so-called Rattenbiss nekrose—rat bite necrosis).

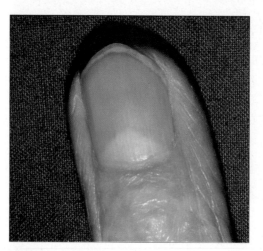

487 Triangular acute angled lunula. This rare autosomal dominant condition (**the nail–patella syndrome**) combines skeletal abnormalities and small or aplastic patellae with nail dystrophy, triangular lunulae and various renal disorders including glomerulonephritis.

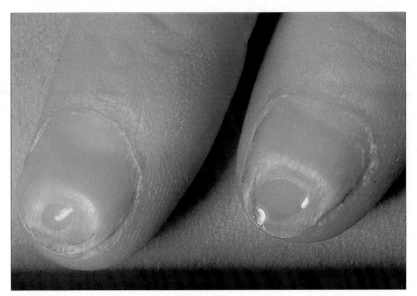

488 Koilonychia—the spoon shaped nail. This flattening of the nail may even be able to hold a drop of fluid. Flat or spooned nails may be normal in young children. It is associated with iron deficiency. It may be seen in growth disorder of the nails in severe illness.

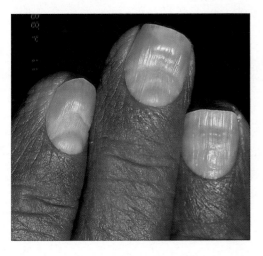

489 Koilonychia in severe illness. This man has recurrent Stevens–Johnson syndrome.

CLUBBING OF THE FINGERS

Clubbing describes the change produced by an increase in tissue volume at the base of the nail, which then becomes spongy to pressure and changes the angle that the nail plate makes with the long axis of the finger (*see* **490**). It is best appreciated by the sensation produced by bouncing the nail on its abnormally spongy bed. As it progresses the finger may become drumstick in profile (*see* **491**, **492**).

Clubbing is seen in:

- Chronic suppurative lung disease.
- Fibrosing lung disease.
- Carcinoma of the bronchus.
- Mesothelioma.
- Heart disease (bacterial endocarditis and cyanotic heart disease).
- Chronic inflammatory bowel disease and liver disease.
- Thyroid acropachy.

The cause remains a puzzle. Many of these diseases are associated with arteriovenous shunts. An attractive explanation is that megakaryocyte fragments fail to be broken up into platelets in the lungs and lodge in the digital vascular capillary bed. These platelet growth factors stimulate vascular growth and clubbing ensues.[97] This would also explain the fact that clubbing is usually less marked in the toes because the fragments are more likely to be broken up during the longer journey to the feet.

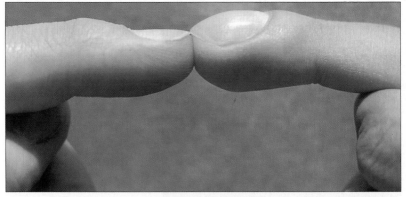

490 Nail clubbing and a normal nail (side view). The normal is on the left.

[97]Dickinson AJ, Martin JF. Megakaryocytes and platelet clumps as the cause of finger nail clubbing. *Lancet*, 1987, **ii**: 1434–5.

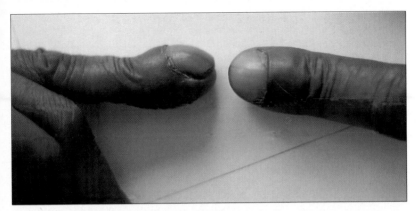

491 Nail clubbing dorsal view. There is beaking and an increase in tissue in a man with bacterial endocarditis.

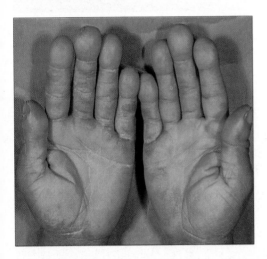

492 Nail clubbing (palmar view). The classic hippocratic nail of drumstick proportions.

In the three examples shown here there is no clue to the cause. The presence of clubbing begs the question... What is the reason? Narrow the possibilities with pertinent questions:

• Do you smoke?
• Do you cough?
• Do you have purulent sputum or diaorrhoea?
• Do you have liver disease?
• Do you have a heart murmur?

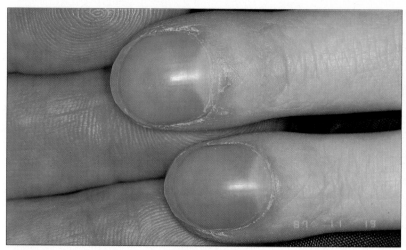

493 Nail clubbing and a normal control. Young cyanosed nails photographed in 1987 (see the date mark). So the cause is more likely to be respiratory than a cardiac anomaly, which would have been corrected surgically. These nails are those of a youth with cystic fibrosis.

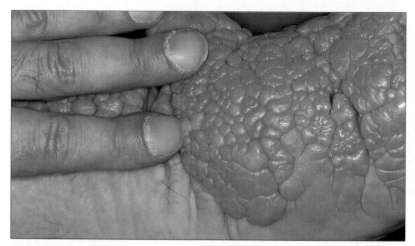

494 Nail clubbing and pretibial myxoedema. The changes of clubbing and gross pretibial myxoedema are extreme. The appearance at the bottom right is more typical (see **742–745**). This is **thyroid acropachyderma** with finger nail clubbing in autoimmune thyroid disease.

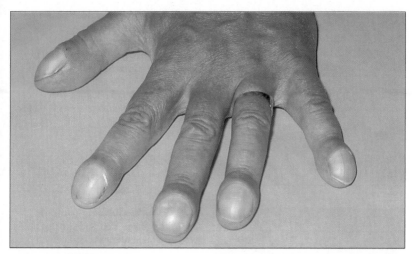

495 Nail clubbing. A heavy cigarette smoker with pain in his lower legs. Not only are his nails clubbed and beaked, but his fingers have taken on a drumstick appearance.

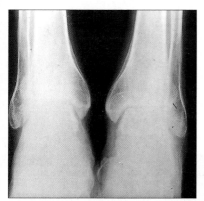

496 Radiograph of the lower leg of the man shown in 495. The periosteal reaction of **hypertrophic pulmonary osteoarthropathy** outlines the cortex and is best seen just above the malleoli. This is associated with carcinoma of the bronchus and suppurative lung disease.

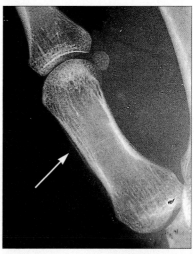

497 Radiograph—of what you see if you know what to look for... Once the change is appreciated then even small degrees of **periosteal reaction** are easily recognised (arrow).

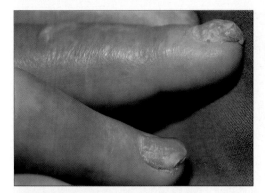

498 Pseudo-clubbing—limited cutaneous scleroderma in progressive systemic sclerosis. The nail grows over the end of the resorbed terminal phalanx. This is not nail clubbing.

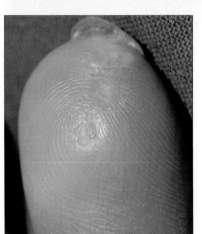

499 Pseudo-clubbing (palmar surface). There is calcinosis at the tip with ulceration and extrusion of material.

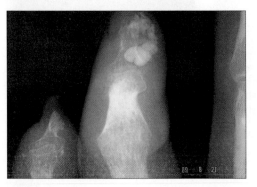

500 Pseudo-clubbing (radiograph of digit). Resorption of the terminal phalanx and subcutaneous calcinosis in **limited cutaneous scleroderma**. Calcinosis may occur in systemic lupus erythematosus and dermatomyositis

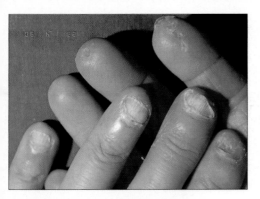

501 Periungual erythema—the CREST syndrome. This patient had **C**alcinosis, **R**aynaud's phenomenon, **E**sophageal involvement, **S**clerodactyly and **T**elangiectasia, which was particularly marked in the periungual area. The fingers are sausage-like.

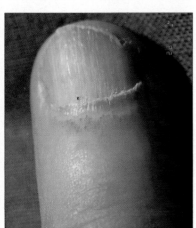

502 Periungual erythema. In close-up, this is seen to be due to dilated capillary loops.

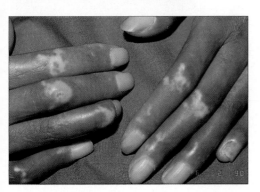

503 The hands in diffuse cutaneous scleroderma. The skin is cold, indurated, hypopigmented, tight and shiny, and there are ulcers over the proximal interphalangeal joints.

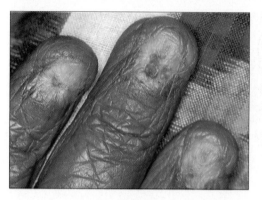

504 The nail pterygium and nail atrophy. The cuticle grows forward over the nail and may lead to total nail atrophy or only a small bit may remain. The epidermis of the dorsal nail fold fuses to the nail bed, and this is seen in digital ischaemia and severe **lichen planus**.

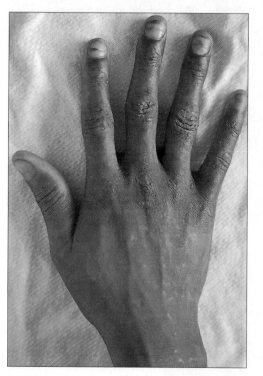

505 Beau's[98] lines (growth arrest lines in systemic disease). The scars of smallpox on the hand and transverse ridges in the nails due to temporary growth arrest at the time of the severe illness. About 0.5–1.2 mm of growth per week dates the illness to about 10 weeks ago. An acute febrile illness or severe disease may lead to arrest of growth and a line or depression in the nail.

[98]Honoré Simon Beau, French physician, 1806–65.

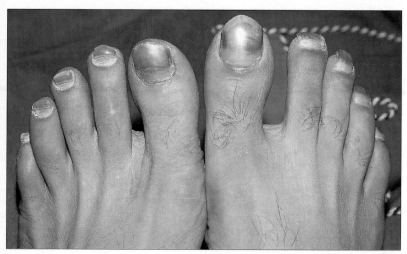

506 Growth arrest lines—local disease and unilateral. Regional insults to a limb may lead to unilateral growth arrest lines. This man had an arterial embolus in the left leg successfully removed about 20 weeks earlier. Toe nail growth rate is about half to one-third of that of the finger nail. The hair growth was also affected.

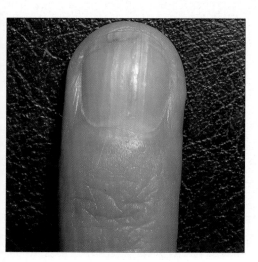

507 Ridging and beading of the nail. This is more common in normal people with advancing age. It is of doubtful significance as a change associated with rheumatoid arthritis.[99]

[99]Hamilton Eric. Nail studies in rheumatoid arthritis. *Ann. Rheum. Dis.*, 1960, **19**: 167.

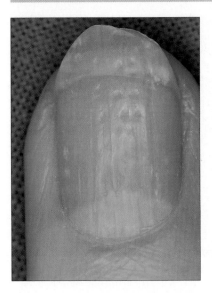

508 Pitting of the nail. This is seen in association with alopecia areata, psoriasis and dermatitis, with larger pits in fungal infections. Minor nail pitting may occur in people with otherwise healthy skin.

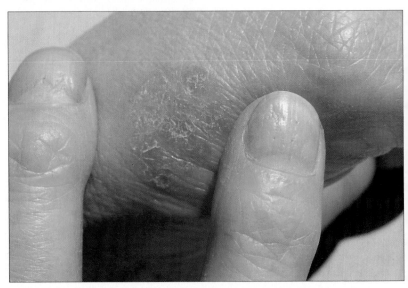

509 Nail pitting in psoriasis. The pits may be sparse on only a few nails or widespread. They are caused by shedding of the weaker parts of the nail keratin, which is laid down in a haphazard way.

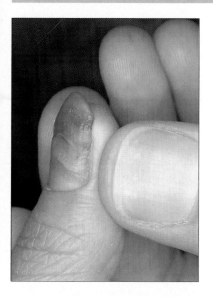

510 Onycholysis of the nail. This is separation of the nail from the bed. In psoriasis it may occur at the free edge (*see* **511**) or start in the centre of the nail and appear as yellow patches called 'oil drops' (*see* **450**). Though a classic change of psoriasis, onycholysis may also be a feature of trauma, fungal infection, Raynaud's phenomenon, thyroid disease, drug reactions and yellow nail syndrome.

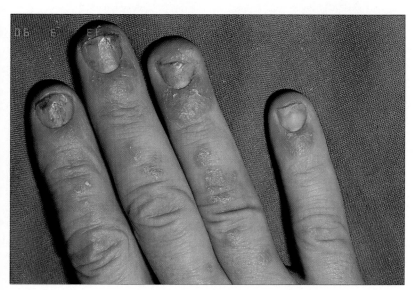

511 Nail changes of psoriasis. This shows the skin plaques of psoriasis, nail pitting, onycholysis and salmon patches. The nail changes may antedate the skin rash.

THE NECK

Many conditions may lead to changes in neck posture. These include:
- Ocular muscle imbalance.
- Muscle overaction as in torticollis, Parkinson's disease, or painful spasm from facet joint displacement, tetanus or meningism secondary to irritation by blood or infection.
- From loss of range of movement by bony fusion.

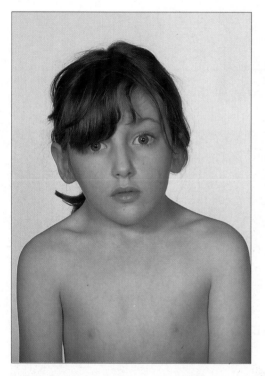

512 The webbed neck. Turner's syndrome,[100] is characterised by a webbed neck, an increased carrying angle at the elbow, amenorrhoea, growth failure and an association with coarctation of the aorta (phenotype XO).

---

[100]Henry Hubert Turner, US endocrinologist, 1892–1970. Turner HH. A syndrome of infantilism, congenital webbed neck, and cubitus valgus. *Endocrinology*, 1938, **23**: 566–74.

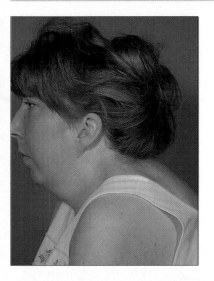

513 The short neck. Klippel–Feil syndrome[101] is characterised by a congenital abnormality in which fusion of the upper cervical vertebrae produces an abnormally short neck. There may be pressure disturbances of the spinal cord or cervical nerve roots.

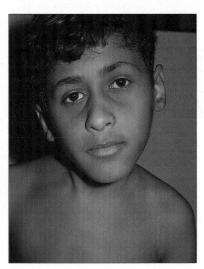

514 Torticollis. Congenital torticollis is produced by contraction of the sternomastoid muscle on the left side with facial asymmetry. **Spasmodic** torticollis is due to dystonic movements, which cause deviation of the head from the neutral position. **Ocular** torticollis may be a compensation for ocular muscle imbalance.

---

[101]Andre Feil, French neurologist, born 1889. Maurice Klippel, French neurologist, 1858–1942. Klippel M, Feil A. Un cas d'absence des vertèbres cervicales avec cage thoracique remantant jusqua'a la base de crâne (cage thoracique cervicale). *Nouv. Icon. Salpêt.*, 1912, **25**: 223–50.

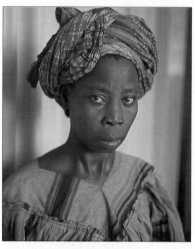

515 Neck stiffness due to muscle spasm. As she sits waiting, note the tense sternomastoids which must be antagonised by the trapezii. This is the muscle stiffness of early **ambulant tetanus**.

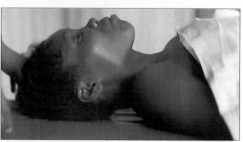

516 Neck stiffness due to muscle spasm. Spasmodic neck retraction and **severe tetanus**. The neck is rigid. Note the gap between the couch and the back of neck. The tense sternomastoids are obvious.

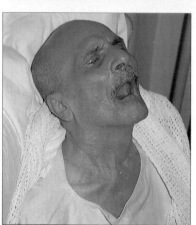

517 Neck stiffness due to meningism. Retraction may occur in meningeal inflammation either due to irritation by blood, acute or chronic meningitis, or disorders of the basal ganglia. If seen in association with a coma, diabetic ketoacidosis, fourth ventricle lesions, severe raised intracranial pressure and tuberculosis must be considered.

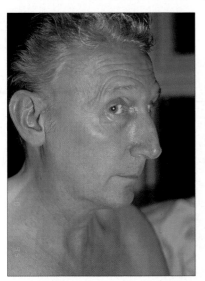

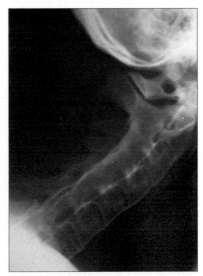

518 Rigid neck due to bony fusion. "Good afternoon" attracts the patient's attention, but only the eyes flick round as the neck is fused by ankylosing spondylitis.

519 Neck radiograph— ankylosing spondylitis. An inflammatory enthesiopathy has lead to syndesmophyte formation and ossification with fusion along the anterior spinal ligament—the **bamboo spine** appearance.

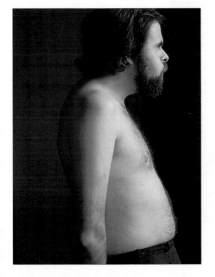

520 Ankylosing spondylitis. The disability of the rigid neck may mean that when standing the visual axis cannot be aligned with the horizontal, even with full extension at the occipito-atlanto-axial joints. Costal expansion is negligible because of fusion of the costovertebral joints. The prominent abdomen is related to the need for diaphragmatic respiration not excess weight.

MIDLINE NECK SWELLINGS

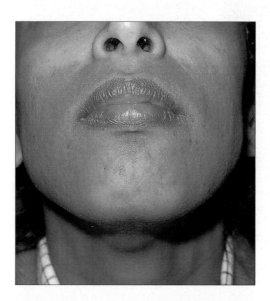

521 Submental. A complaint of a lump under the chin and perioral rash. The submental lymph gland is a midline structure immediately anterior to the hyoid bone and must be differentiated from a thyroglossal sinus (*see* **522**).

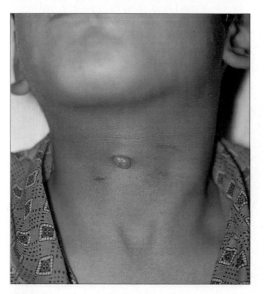

522 A thyroglossal sinus. A thyroglossal cyst and sinus are remnants of the thyroglossal duct. The cyst moves on swallowing and tongue protrusion and may be present anywhere from the base of the tongue around the hyoid to the base of the neck.

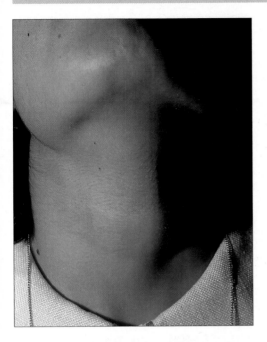

523 The midline thyroid.
The appearance of this central midline swelling is that of a thyroglossal cyst and may even move on tongue protrusion. It is important before excising an apparent thyroglossal cyst to ensure that this is not the only thyroid tissue that the patient has. A radioiodine scan of the neck showed that there was no other functioning thyroid tissue present, confirming the midline thyroid.

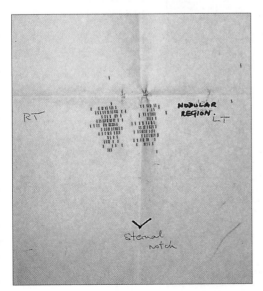

524 Midline thyroid—Iodine[131] uptake scan.
The midline thyroid in **523** is confirmed by a radioiodine scan.

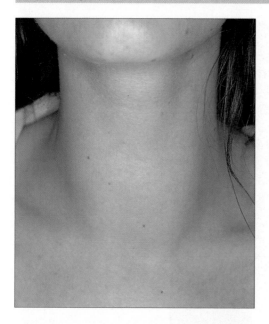

525 The normal thyroid.
This moves on swallowing.

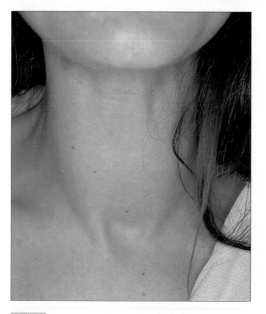

526 The normal thyroid on swallowing. It moves because it is attached to the thyroid cartilage.

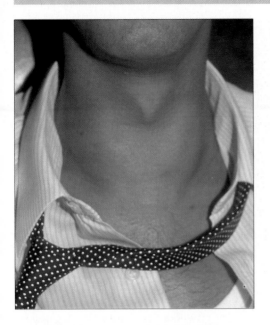

527 Enlarged thyrotoxic gland. The thyroid is very obvious when enlarged.

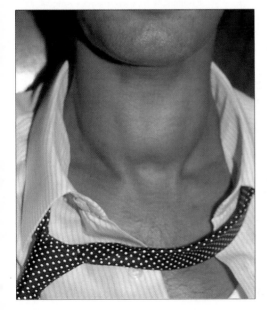

528 Enlarged thyrotoxic gland on swallowing. The enlarged gland can be assessed on swallowing. The swelling may be noted during a consultation for an unrelated problem.

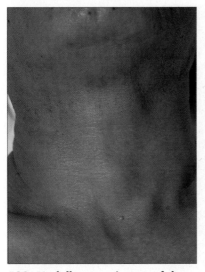

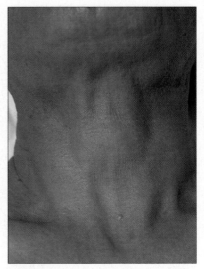

529 Medullary carcinoma of the thyroid and attached glands. This man complained of recent sciatic pain. As the leg was examined and straight leg raising assessed, a glance at his face caught the thyroid and gland on the left as they moved on swallowing (*see* **530**).

530 Medullary carcinoma of the thyroid and movement on swallowing. The thyroid and gland on the left side moved on swallowing. A medullary carcinoma of thyroid.

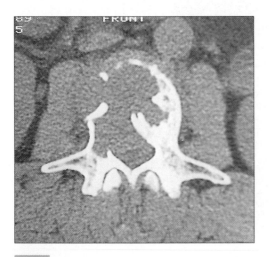

531 Computerised tomographic scan of the lumbar vertebra of the patient shown in 530. Metastases are seen in the lumbar spine.

DIFFERENTIAL DIAGNOSIS OF LATERAL SWELLINGS IN THE NECK

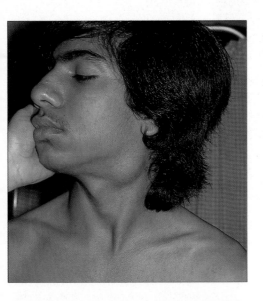

532 The branchial cyst.
Peeping from behind the upper third of the sternomastoid muscle, this is smooth and painless. It must be differentiated from a metastatic lymph gland, a neurofibroma and a lipoma. Enlargement of the laryngeal saccule—a laryngocoele—into the neck between the thyroid and hyoid cartilages may be seen in wind instrument players.

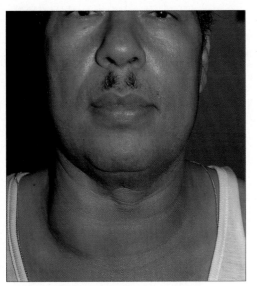

533 A right carotid aneurysm. Pulsation in the neck may be arterial or venous. Carotid pulsation may be due to a kinked carotid artery, often on the right, or a carotid aneurysm. The sac may predispose to clot formation and subsequent emboli.

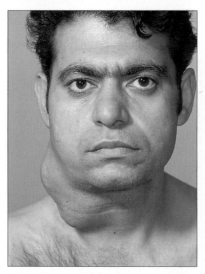

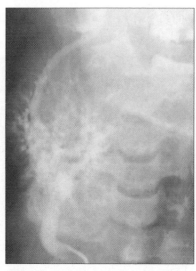

534 The carotid body tumour. This may be felt deeper than a branchial cyst posterior to the sternomastoid and in its lower two-thirds.

535 Carotid body tumour (angiogram). It is solid and at the bifurcation of the common carotid artery. It does not vary in size and is not necessarily pulsatile. There may be a bruit. It can be moved from side to side, but not vertically.

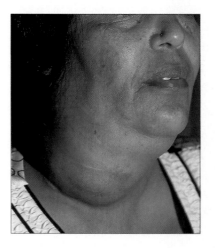

536 Cystic hygroma.[102] This is a fluctuant and brightly transilluminating multilocular lymphangiomatous swelling. It is liable to recurrent infection. These episodes have been treated with counter-irritation using a red hot iron—the burn marks can be seen as horizontal scars on the neck.

[102]Cystic hygroma. *Lancet*, 1990, 335 8688: 511–12.

INFECTION

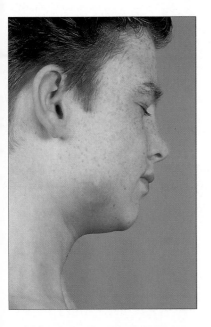

537 Cat scratch disease. Cellulitis in the neck with associated tender suppurative regional lymphadenopathy developed about two weeks after a scratch from a cat. This is caused by the organism *Bartonella henselae*, a gram-negative rod. Cutaneous bacillary angiomatosis in human immunodeficiency virus (HIV)-positive individuals is clinically similar to Kaposi's sarcoma and is related to cats and *Bartonella henselae* and *B. quintana*.

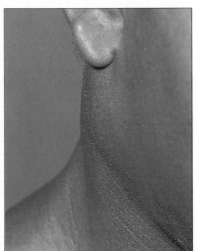

538 The apex of the anterior triangle and tuberculosis. Enlargement of the lymph gland in the upper cervical chain must be distinguished from swelling around the ear due to, for example, a sebaceous cyst or tumour. The lymph gland is seen at the upper border of the sternomastoid.

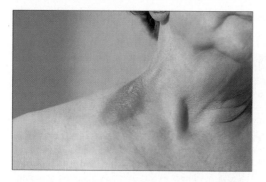

539 The cold abscess—the collar stud abscess. Sinus formation and incipient ulceration with a characteristic lividity is typical of the collar stud abscess in which the superficial caseous material communicates with a deeper collection through the fascia in the neck.

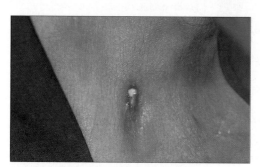

540 Caseous material at the sinus orifice. Pressure on the abscess may extrude caseous material from the sinus.

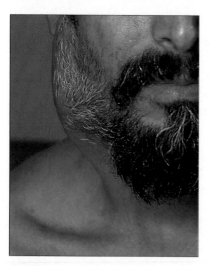

541 Lymphoma. This man has a six-week story of fever, weight loss and a swelling in his neck. Hodgkin's[103] disease usually presents with enlargement of lymphatic tissue—often glands in the neck or axillae—and the physical consequences of such expansion with impaired function of the immune system. Non-specific B cell symptoms of weight loss and night sweats may indicate a more serious prognosis.

[103]Thomas Hodgkin, English physician, 1798–1866. Hodgkin T. On some morbid appearances of the absorbent glands and spleen. *Med. Chir. Tr.* (London), 1832, **17**: 68–114.

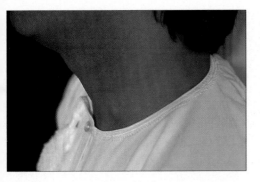

542 The epileptic fit. This man complained of a recent onset of nocturnal enuresis and while sitting in the consulting room had a grand mal epileptic fit. The lump at his collar had been seen, but its significance became clear when many small subcutaneous lumps were then found on examination. The lump on the neck was biopsied (*see* **543**).

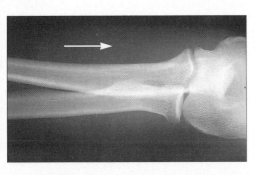

543 Chitinous hooks on biopsy and radiograph of a calcified palpable nodule in the arm. The chitinous hooks of a scolex show up in partially polarised light. The diagnosis is **cerebral cysticercosis**—an infection with the larval stage of *Taenia solium*, which is normally found in pigs! Of new epileptics in areas harbouring *T. solium*, only 20% may have such nodules. The nodules may show up on radiological examination. The calcified cyst is seen adjacent to the ulna. This is muscular cysticercosis. Cysticercosis may also affect the eye.

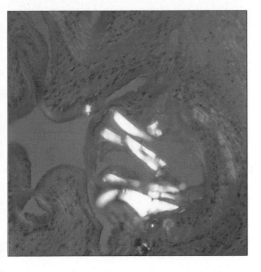

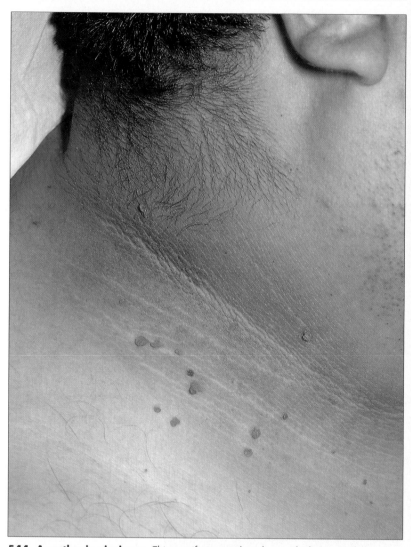

544 Acanthosis nigricans. This manifests as velvety-brown thickening with warty excrescences affecting the skin of the hands and skin folds in the axillae, groins, neck and at mucocutaneous junctions. It is benign when associated with obesity, diabetes mellitus, acromegaly and polycystic ovary syndrome—a clinical marker of insulin resistance and hyperinsulinism. It is malign in an older age group when it affects the lips, face and hands and may indicate an underlying adenocarcinoma.

VENOUS DISTENSION IN THE NECK

A detailed analysis of the venous waves: a (from atrial contraction), c (transmitted from the carotid artery), v (reflecting tricuspid closure and therefore atrial filling), and the pressure changes these venous waves reflect assumes the ability to see the elevated column of blood in the first place. The prerequisites are:

- An oblique light.
- A relaxed patient lying supported at an angle that allows the vein to fill.
- A vein oscillating with breathing and the heart beat that varies with hepatic pressure.

Know where to look, note the change with breathing and hepatic compression on the venous column, and differentiate between a nerve, the external and internal jugular veins and arterial pulsation by observation, palpation and timing the venous pulse.

Freely fluctuating venous distension

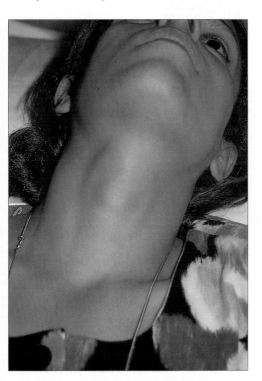

545 The internal jugular vein. This is the best manometer for venous pressure assessment. It is straight, communicates without valves with the right atrium, and reflects increased right atrial pressure. It lies medial and deep to the sternomastoid muscle running upwards from behind the sternoclavicular joint to the angle of the jaw. In normal people the vertical height from the top of the column to the angle is usually less than 3 cm, while the atrium lies 5 cm below the angle so that there is therefore 8 cm of blood column. In this woman the pressure is elevated, being 10 cm above the sternal angle.

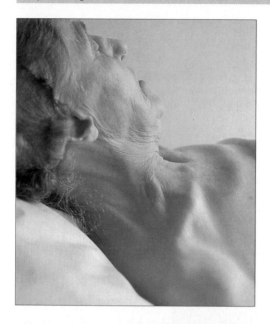

546 The external jugular vein. Lying superficial to the sternomastoid and running obliquely across it, the external jugular vein is easier to see than the internal jugular vein, but prone to kinking and may mislead the unwary.

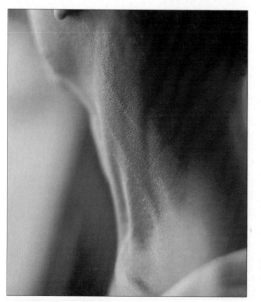

547 Hypertrophic nerves. The hypertrophied greater auricular nerve running across the sternomastoid muscle in **tuberculoid leprosy**. The angle that the nerve makes with the muscle is quite different to that of the external jugular vein. Thickened nerves may occur in hypertrophic neuropathies, sarcoidosis, neoplasms, reticuloses and amyloidosis. Neurofibromatosis and the effect of trauma may also lead to thick nerves.

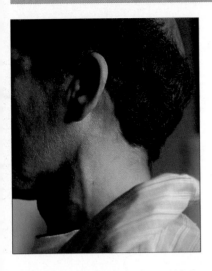

548 Tricuspid incompetence. This man presented with gross cardiac failure and functional tricuspid incompetence due to cardiac dilatation of the valve ring. The top of the venous column in the external jugular vein is above the angle of the jaw.

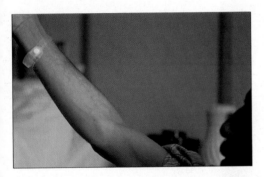

549 The head of pressure in the arm of the man shown in 548. The top of the venous column can be made to appear when the arm is held above the head (*see* **550**). Here the veins are empty.

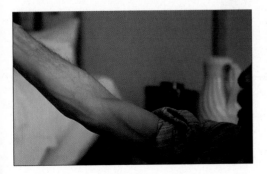

550 The head of pressure in the arm of the man shown in 548 and 549. As the arm is slowly lowered and the vein fills the top of the column becomes visible.

Fixed venous distension

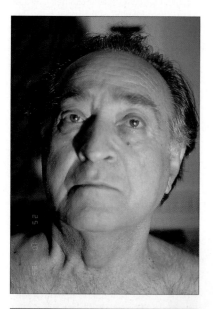

551 Partial mediastinal obstruction before radiotherapy.
Large metastatic glands from bronchial carcinoma obstruct the venous drainage on the right side of the neck. No pulsation is transmitted.

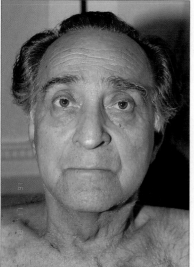

552 Partial mediastinal obstruction after radiotherapy.
Note the right mediastinoscopy scar and the radiotherapy-marking pencil. His face is also thinner than in **551** and reflects the wasting of progressive malignant disease.

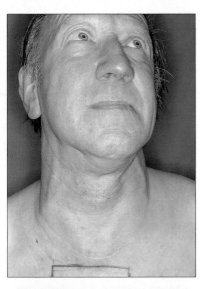

553 Superior mediastinal obstruction distended neck veins.
Once the block to venous return from the head and neck is bilateral the appearance of superior mediastinal obstruction develops. At first bilateral fixed venous distension is seen. There is a scar in the suprasternal notch due to an old thyroid operation.

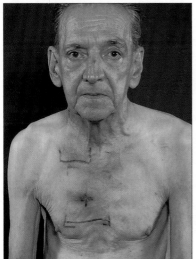

554 Superior mediastinal obstruction plethora. Plethora with ocular suffusion accompanies the venous engorgement.

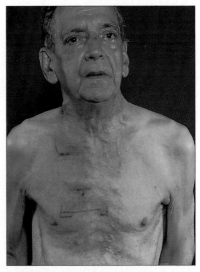

555 Superior mediastinal obstruction. Despite the radiotherapy to the mediastinum the obstruction has increased, plethora is marked and collateral veins appear on the chest.

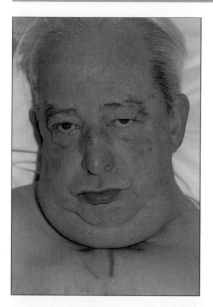

556 Conjunctiveal injection in superior mediastinal obstruction. The face becomes swollen and cyanosed. There is conjunctival injection from venous engorgement.

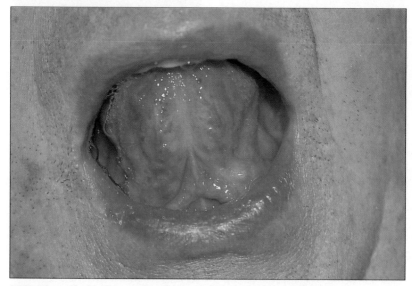

557 Distended veins under the tongue in superior mediastinal obstruction. Under the tongue distended veins are also visible.

THE CHEST

Occupation may be relevant in chest disease. Clues may abound.

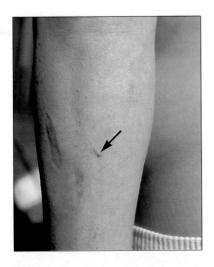

558 The tattoo of coal mining. This man presented with cough and breathlessness. The intradermal implantation of coal in a man who gave up coal mining as an occupation long ago gives a clue to the cause of his fibrotic lung disease (arrow).

The shape on inspection and inequality of movement on palpation are valuable pointers to underlying pathology.

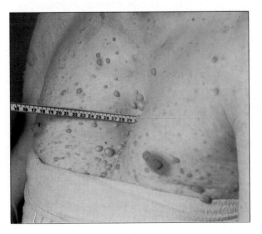

559 Pectus excavatum. This is a congenital anomaly - it may cause displacement of the apex beat and thus an apparently enlarged heart on the chest xray. A murmur may be heard. It is not significant. The skin shows multiple neurofibromata (neurofibromatosis type 1, see **40**). Look at the hands for arachnodactyly and the palate (**423a, 423b**) for Marfan's syndrome, which may be present.

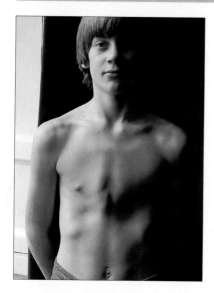

560 Pectus carinatus. This is also called pigeon chest and is common. The prominent sternum may be congenital or a legacy of childhood rickets or asthma. The sulcus—Harrison's sulcus[104]—on the lower aspect of the chest may be caused by indrawing of the ribs by muscle attachments in asthma.

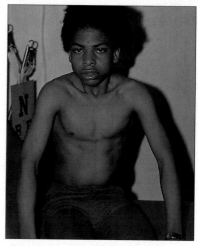

562 Acute bronchial asthma. This youth needs to place his hands on the couch to fix his shoulder girdle and then use his pectorals and sternomastoids as accessory muscles of respiration. His alae nasi are flaring in concert. Other patterns of respiration depend on changes in rhythmn and rate. An increase in rate is always important, but must be observed circumspectly. The shallow breathing may be due to pain, sighing respirations may reflect acidosis, and deep gasping hyperventilation, stress. Inability to lie flat suggests oedema of the lungs, and pursed lip breathing, airflow obstruction. Periods of apnoea may accompany brain stem dysfunction.

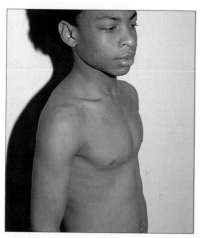

561 Chronic bronchial asthma. This youth with chronic bronchial asthma has prominent pectoral muscle and an early pigeon chest.

[104]Edwin Harrison, English physician at St. Marylebone Infirmary, London, 1779–1847.

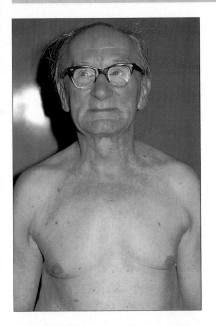

563 The barrel chest. The increase in volume of the chest leads to this appearance, and is related to the increased volume of the lungs in emphysema. The ribs are lifted to the horizontal in an inspiratory position and breathing may be diaphragmatic and expansion poor. The areas of cardiac dullness and hepatic dullness may be diminished as the voluminous lungs encroach upon them.

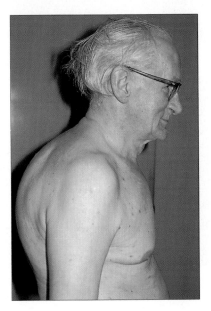

564 The barrel chest (lateral view). The increase in the anteroposterior diameter leads to the barrel chest. This man also has a kyphosis produced by wedging of the thoracic vertebrae, which may be marked in postmenopausal women, leading to the 'dowager's hump'.

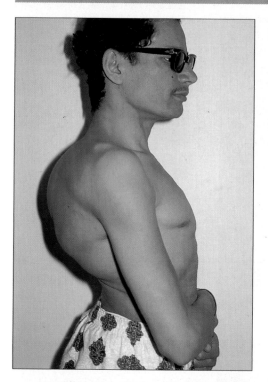

565 The gibbus.[105] There is vertical loss of height of the thoracic spine with angulation due to vertebral collapse from tuberculous osteomyelitis.

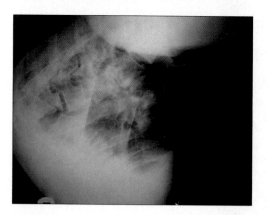

566 The gibbus (chest radiograph). On the lateral chest radiograph the acute angulation of the gibbus due to the vertebral collapse reduces the vital capacity and the respiratory reserve.

[105]Etymology: latin, *gibbus*, *gibbosus*, hump, hump backed.

THE ASYMMETRICAL CHEST

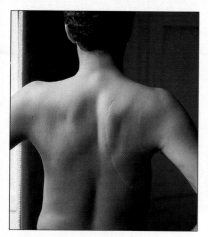

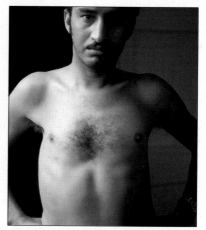

567 The thoracoplasty. Scars may be a clue to previous disease. The deformity produced by thoracoplasty for tuberculosis may be minimal from the back.

568 The thoracoplasty. However, the collapse of the apex of the lung produced by pushing in the rib cage can be clearly seen in the right axillary region from the front.

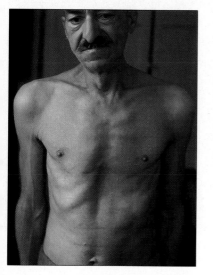

569 Pulmonary fibrosis and depression of the rib cage. There is flattening of the left chest wall and diminished expansion. Scoliosis of the spine with its rotatory component throws part of the chest into prominence and the anterior part on the side of the convexity will appear flattened. If no scoliosis exists then flattening may indicate long-standing unilateral pulmonary disease, usually pulmonary fibrosis, rather than collapse. There is usually mediastinal shift.

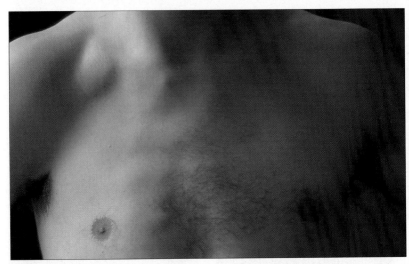

570 Congenital failure of development of pectoralis major—1. Apparent
flattening may be due to change in the muscles of the chest wall. Here pectoralis major
is rudimentary from birth.

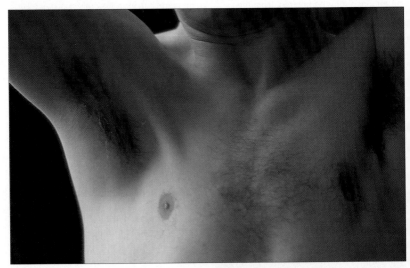

571 Congenital failure of development of pectoralis major—2. Only a
small slip of muscle is seen on abduction of the arm.

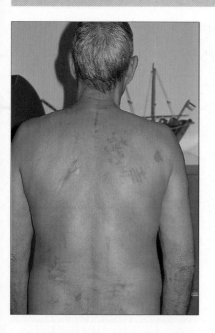

572 Back pain treatment. This is not decorative tattooing. The deduction is recurrent low back and shoulder pains treated with counter-irritation.

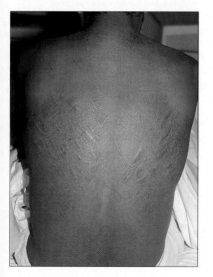

573 Religious flagellation. These scars in a devout Shiite Muslim reflect self flagellation at a period of religious mourning[106] in Moharram, the first month of the Muslim year of 30 days. Their diagonal direction reflects the cut of the lash as it is flicked over each shoulder.

---

[106]In memory of the assassination of Ali, Mohammed's cousin and son-in-law, and his son Hussain.

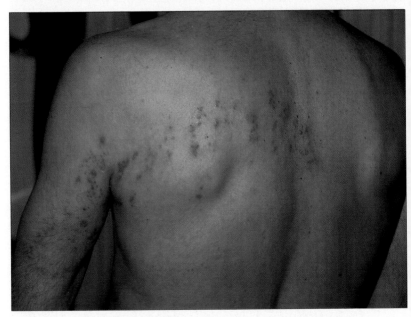

574 Herpes zoster (shingles[107]). In the middle-aged person with waning immunity, in haematological malignancy and in immunosuppression (induced by drugs or human immunodeficiency virus), a childhood infection with herpes zoster/varicella virus may reactivate. Here the third thoracic dermatome is involved. The inflammatory process is based on the dormant infection in the dorsal root ganglion. Pain and hyperalgesia first occur in the area supplied by the affected root and are followed later by the vesicular rash, which maps the dermatome. If spread occurs back to the anterior horn cells, motor weakness may follow in the same segment. It is easy to diagnose on the trunk and face, but diagnosis is less easy on the limb where the anatomical distribution may not be immediately appreciated. In the stage before a rash the dysaesthesiae can be mapped out and a diagnosis made before the rash is clear-cut.

---

[107]Etymology: latin, *cingulus, cingulum*, girdle, *cingere*, gird; arabic, *hizzam al nari*, 'belt of fire'; norwegian, '*a belt of roses from hell.*'

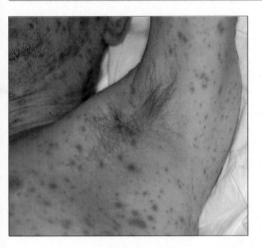

575 Varicella—chicken-pox. This actor was in a long-running play on Broadway, New York in the 1980s. He developed severe chickenpox while in hospital for a hernia repair in the 1990s. The fluid-filled vesicles on a red base are interspersed with macules and papules of the eruption in the initial phases. In the adult the illness may lead to severe systemic upset and have a more prolonged course in the immunocompromised individual with human immunodeficiency virus.

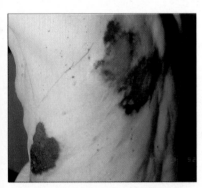

576 Haemorrhagic herpes zoster (purpura fulminans). This may develop at about the sixth day of the rash and is a serious complication that also occurs in chickenpox. Here it is mimicked by bleeding into the zoster in this man who has been anticoagulated with warfarin.

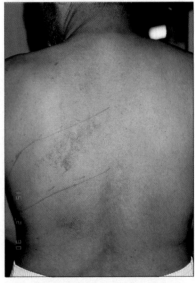

577 Postherpetic hyperaesthesia and pigmentation. Once resolved, scarring may remain with residual hyperalgesia, which has been mapped with a pin, outlining the fourth thoracic dermatome.

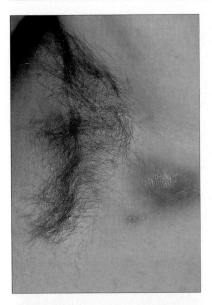

578 Axilla—hidradenitis suppurativa. A chronic inflammatory condition of apocrine gland follicle-bearing skin. It may affect the axillae and perineal skin, and is often due to anaerobic infection. It may be associated with Crohn's disease and be complicated by an inflammatory arthropathy or pyoderma gangrenosum.

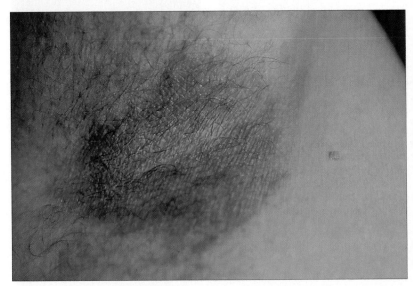

579 Erythrasma of the axilla. Pigmentation of the axillae or groins may be due to superficial skin infection with a *Corynebacterium*.

580 The axilla of 579 illuminated by ultraviolet light. Examination under ultraviolet light shows the characteristic coral-red fluorescence. In hot climates it may lead to intractable itching.

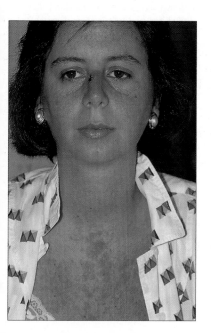

581 Photosensitivity rashes and the V of the neck line. A day of sun bathing led to cutaneous erythema on light-exposed areas. The relationship of the rash to sunlight is easily appreciated because it is the malar area that is affected, as in sunburn, and it is the open neckline that demonstrates the V-like rash. This is **systemic lupus erythematosus** with a malar rash and a macular erythema in the neckline. A skin biopsy has been performed. Facial oedema may be a feature.

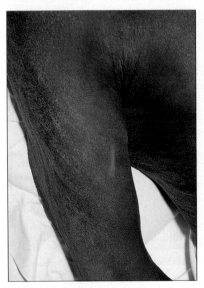

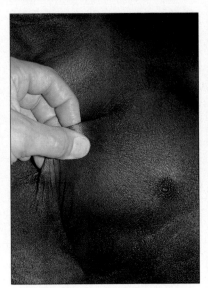

582 Weight loss. Recent weight loss is often easily appreciated in the skin of the upper chest and arms.

583 Weight loss on the chest—picking up the skin. The skin is lax, easily lifted and falls in folds. If the individual is dehydrated it may remain standing in folds when released because the tissue turgor is reduced.

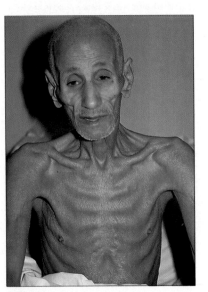

584 Weight loss. In the investigation of weight loss the single most helpful investigation may be the chest radiograph. When the loss is long-standing subcutaneous fat disappears and the bones are visible. This old man has inadequate intake, yet his eyes are bright in contrast to the appearance of cachexia (*see* **141**). There is always a risk of pressure sores.

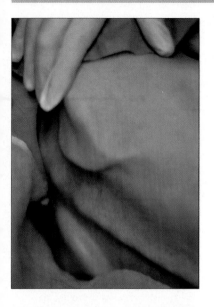

585 Weight loss and bony points.
If the patient is ill and immobile and the body weight is concentrated on bony prominences, breakdown is due to a combination of pressure and shearing force, complicated by impaired sensation and circulation. It is vital to realise that a decubitus[108] ulcer may occur in hours—even while waiting in an accident and emergency department on a hard trolley.

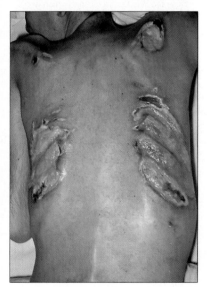

586 Pressure sores over ribs and scapulae.
Decubitus ulcers can lead to pressure sores exposing bone. These sores are due to neglect; note the points where they have occurred. Always check these areas—the sacrum, trochanters, medial condyles, femurs, heels and malleoli—in any debilitated patient, particularly if the ward is understaffed. The earliest sign of redness may be picked up before the skin breaks.

---

[108]Etymology: latin, *decumbere, decumbent,* lie down.

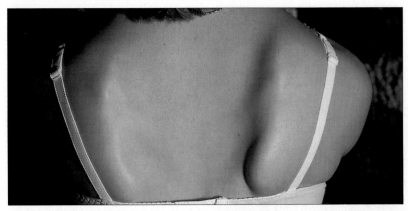

587 Isolated winging of the scapula. When prominent at rest and on arm abduction, consider middle trapezius weakness due to a lesion of the spinal accessory nerve. If brought out on forward flexion of the arm, as in leaning against a wall on the outstretched hands, which flings the isolated winged scapula into prominence, the presumed cause is an isolated infective lesion of the nerve to serratus anterior (C5,6,7), as in motor herpes zoster. In muscle disease, such as facioscapulohumeral muscular dystrophy, the inferior medial edge of the scapula juts out first because the base of the crane (which has the arm boom attached) is not fixed when the arm is lifted away from the body.

SWELLINGS OF THE CHEST WALL

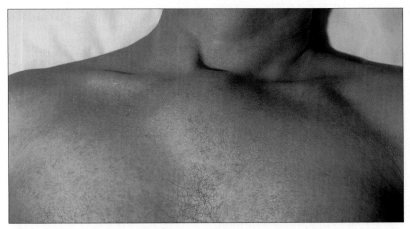

588 Swelling of the manubrium and differential diagnosis. In subcutaneous tissues the swelling will be a lipoma, while if swelling is in the sternum it will be a bony tumour or plasmacytoma. A pulsatile swelling from within will be an eroding aortic aneurysm.

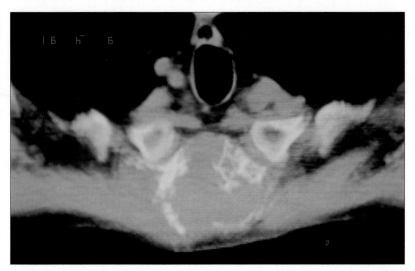

589 Plasmacytoma (computerised tomographic scan). The scan reveals the expanding solitary lytic lesion of a plasmacytoma.

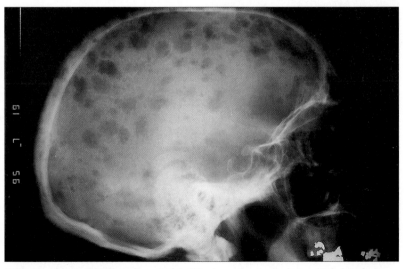

590 Myeloma (skull radiograph). This shows the similar but multiple lytic lesions of disseminated myeloma.

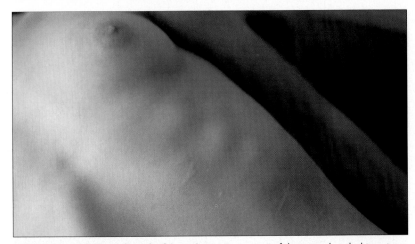

591 Enlarged costochondral junctions. Expansion of the costochondral junction reflects a growth abnormality, due to either a failure of mineralisation in vitamin D deficiency with the expanded osteoid producing a **rickety rosary**, or **acromegaly**. They may act as a biological marker of previous or current growth hormone excess.[109]

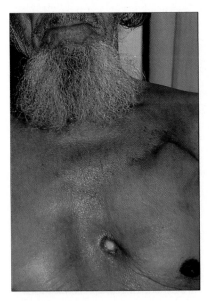

592 The chest sinus. When due to a neglected empyema (empyema necessitatis) a discharging sinus anywhere on the chest wall may be preceded by a swelling with a cough impulse. Here, a tuberculous infection has occurred in the glands of the internal mammary chain and has pointed lateral to the sternum. The caseous material has exuded producing a situation comparable to that of the collar stud abscess in the neck (*see* **539**). This man has a pacemaker in the upper chest.

---

[109]Ibbertson N *et al.* The acromegaly rosary. *Lancet*, 1991, **337**(8734):154–6.

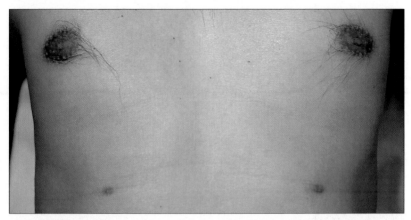

593 A Japanese electronics engineer with bilateral accessory nipples. The supernumerary nipple may occur anywhere along a line from the shoulder to the hip. In the twentieth century it has little significance. In the past it was one stigma of witchcraft and was used to confirm an allegation of witchcraft because it showed that the accused suckled a familiar[110] who acted as the channel for communication with Satan. In the Salem, Massachusetts witch trials in 1692–3, 148 women and 56 men were accused of witchcraft.[111] Accessory nipples are seen in up to 2.5% of people, and some were put to death on such confirmatory evidence.[112]

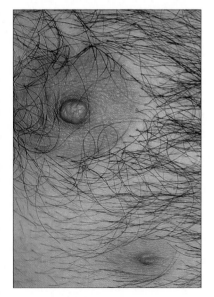

594 The accessory nipple. The extra nipple or nipples vary from a pigmented macule to a nipple with an areola.

---

[110]In full—familiar spirit—a demon supposedly attending and obeying a witch.
[111]Demos JP. Underlying themes in witchcraft of seventeenth century New England. *American Historical Review*, LXXXIV (1979): 317–46.
[112]If you have one, don't indulge in time travel back to the seventeenth century, for you risk burning at a stake or worse!

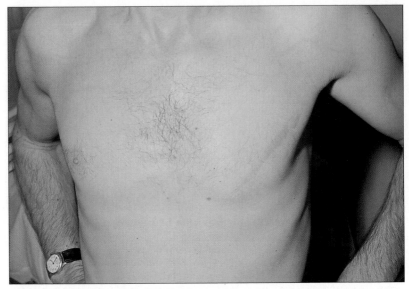

595 A unilateral chest scar in a male. A male with a mastectomy scar. It is important to appreciate the potential significance of such a scar to the presenting complaint. Breast cancer is uncommon in the male, but more frequent in XXY phenotypes.

GYNAECOMASTIA (BENIGN MALE BREAST ENLARGEMENT)

Gynaecomastia may be unilateral or bilateral and appears if there is a change in the ratio of free oestrogen to free androgen.

- It occurs physiologically at puberty and in the elderly male with declining Leydig cell function.
- In pseudogynaecomastia due to obesity ('gynosity') or tumours there is no true increase in glandular tissue.
- Oestrogens, taken either deliberately or unintentionally, as well as digitalis acting as an oestrogen like substance, and drugs that cause testosterone suppression such as spironolactone and cimetidine or have an antiandrogen effect, may lead to the development of excess glandular tissue.

In the majority of cases, the cause is a drug, an excess of oestrogen or a decrease in testosterone levels. Increased oestrogen may be due to a testicular or bronchial tumour, an adrenal carcinoma or liver disease.

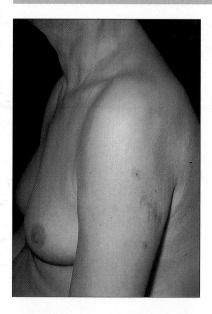

596 Gynaecomastia. The presence of two vascular spider naevi on the arm suggest a diagnosis of liver cirrhosis.

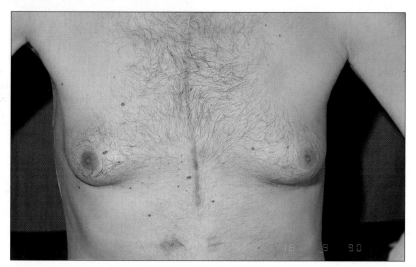

597 Gynaecomastia with a sternal scar. Gynaecomastia and a recent median sternotomy. Heart disease treated with digoxin and diuretics (including **spironolactone**) led to breast enlargement.

287

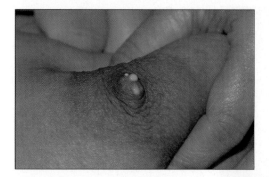

598 Galactorrhoea. This is a discharge of milk in the absence of parturition. It may occur in either sex and is a manifestation of hyperprolactinaemia.

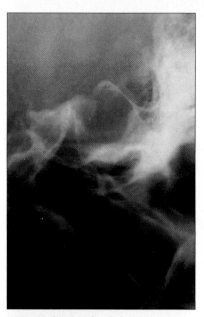

599 Radiograph of the pituitary fossa of the man shown in 598. The man has galactorrhoea related to a pituitary tumour, which has caused enlargement of the pituitary fossa.

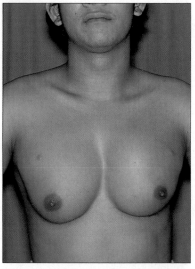

600 Breathlessness in a juvenile. A very distressed young person was admitted as an emergency with breathlessness. The chest radiograph showed bilateral 'bat's wing' shadows over the middle zones. Diuretics were administered with *very* good effect. The hyperventilation subsided. On the early morning ward round, the house officer was chastened to be shown that the lung shadows were due to breast prostheses in an overwrought and overbreathing transvestite.

THE ABDOMEN

Examination of the abdomen begins with a glance at the chest and palpation of the supraclavicular fossae followed by palpation of the abdomen while watching the facial expression. Other clues may be evident, for example the belt can be used as an objective witness to gauge weight change when no record is kept.

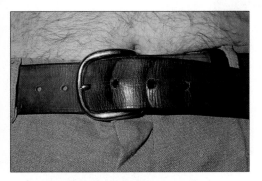

601 Belt notch markings and their significance. This man is an Offshore Construction Manager of an oil platform in the North Sea—a sedentary job for half the day and then walking all around an oil installation for the remainder. The belt was loosened for sitting and tightened for doing his rounds, so there are two marks of equal intensity reflecting sitting and standing. The second pair reflects deliberate weight loss following his company periodic health check-up, but as he was back onshore, his whole day was spent sitting and the need to tighten it while standing was minimal.

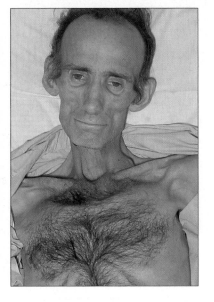

602 Troisier's[113] sign. This is an enlarged lymph node in the left supraclavicular triangle due to regional spread from a carcinoma of the stomach or testis. It is easily overlooked if it is small and tucked behind the head of the clavicle.

[113]Charles Emile Troisier, French physician, 1848–1919.

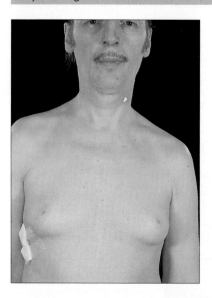

603 The chest with gynaecomastia. It is wise to look at the chest when examining the abdomen. Gynaecomastia, spider naevi on the chin and left upper chest and a liver biopsy dressing all add up to an abdominal problem—cirrhosis of the liver.

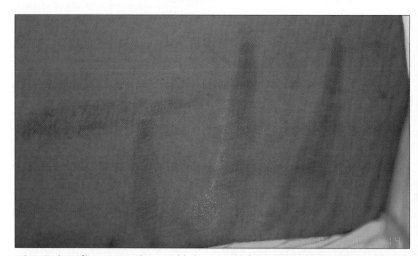

604 Striae distensae. These visible linear scars form in skin that has been damaged by stretching forces in areas where there has been a particular and rapid increase in bulk. They are common in adolescence across the thighs and lumbosacral areas, over the lower abdomen and breasts in pregnancy (striae gravidarum) and on the shoulders in young weight lifters. They are also seen in Cushing's syndrome and with systemic steroid therapy. Initially striae are raised and irritable and then become smooth and livid.

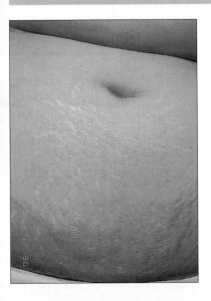

605 Striae gravidarum. Ultimately striae become white.

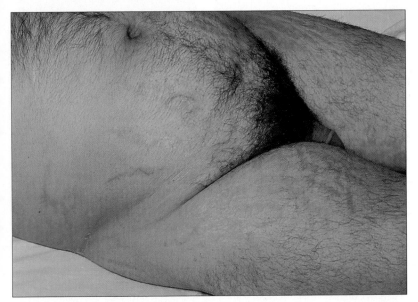

606 Striae in Cushing's syndrome. The striae may be conspicuous and even affect the face. When due to topical corticosteroid therapy they appear at the site of application.

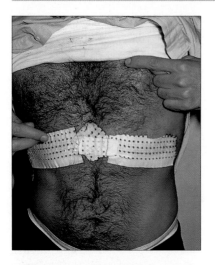

607 Abdominal pain—"my pain is here!" Modern self-medication—the belladonna plaster used as a counter irritant outlines the radiation of gall bladder colic from the epigastrium along the costal margins.

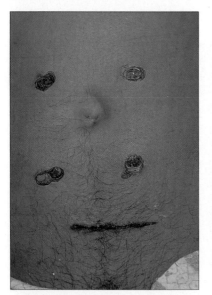

608 Abdominal pain—"my pain is here!" Traditional medication—treatment by cautery used as counter-irritation. The cautery site may be a standard one used for abdominal pain with no localising value.

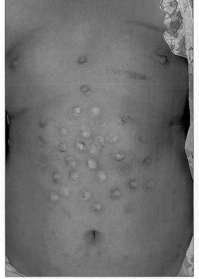

609 Abdominal pain and the history from the abdominal scars. Sometimes fresh and old cautery scars (*see* **608**) tell a story of recurrent discomfort.

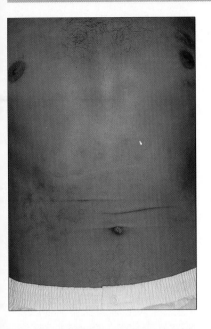

610 Right upper quadrant pain— the cautery and gallstones.
Sometimes cautery scars point directly to the site of maximal pain in gall stone colic.

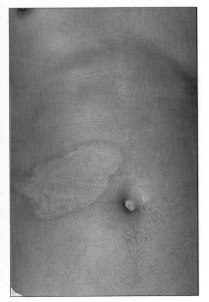

611 Right upper quadrant scar and the hot water bottle. The use of heat as counter-irritation may lead to a burn.

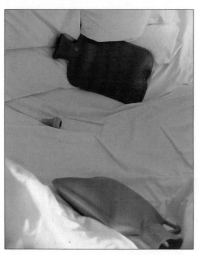

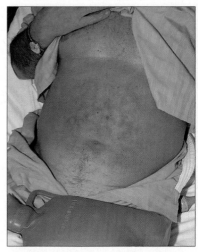

612 Examination of the bed 1–no patient. Pain at specific sites has certain characteristics. The bed rest is raised[114] and a hot water bottle as a heat source is placed to the lower back, while another hot water bottle has been tossed aside.[115]

613 Examination of the bed 2– erythema ab igne. The patient is back from the latrines. The heat application is of such long-standing that the changes of erythema ab igne[116] are seen in the epigastrium.

614 Examination of the bed 3–the back. As the pain spreads through into the back another heat source leads to erythema in the small of the back. This is a characteristic story of **retroperitoneal pain** and **carcinoma of the pancreas**.

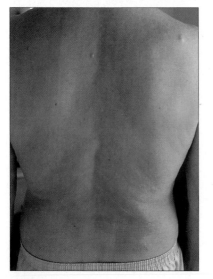

---

[114]The patient prefers to sit up—the pain is better if the abdomen is flexed.
[115]This suggests that the pain felt in the abdomen goes through to the back. The pain is worsened by lying flat and/or relieved by doubling up.
[116]Literally 'redness from the fire'—a skin change induced by chronic application of heat and seen on the legs from radiant heat of a fire as well as from a heatpad. The question to ask is "why does the individual feel the cold"? Perhaps they have no heating due to poverty or they feel the cold excessively and huddle to the fire to keep warm— an important sign of hypothyroidism.

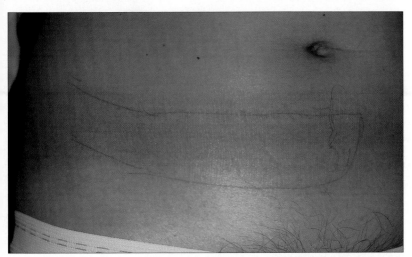

615 Abdominal pain and hyperaesthesiae (a pitfall). Right iliac fossa pain may be due to peritoneal irritation, but pain may precede a herpes zoster rash. The area of changed sensation (11th thoracic dermatome) can be mapped with a sharp instrument.

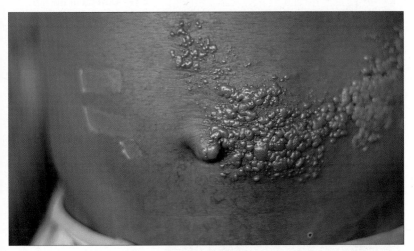

616 Herpes zoster. The fully developed rash is limited to one (10th thoracic) dermatome, stops at the midline and affects half the small umbilical hernia. The normal umbilicus is inverted. Eversion may be due to a hernia or an increase in abdominal contents by fluid, flatus, viscera or tumour. This small central weakness is common in the protein-deficient African child and may also become apparent when filled with ascites.

THE UMBILICUS

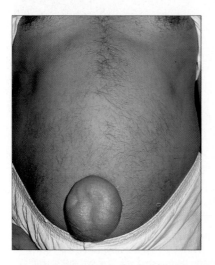

617 Umbilical hernia (irreducible).
Though obvious clinically this may cause confusion when seen on a plain abdominal radiograph as a circular gas-containing shadow in the centre of the film.

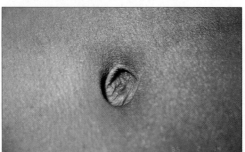

618 Umbilical hernia (lying flat). Abdominal ascites may fill a small hernia of the umbilicus (*see* **619**).

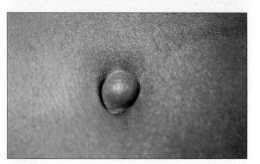

619 Umbilical hernia full of ascitic fluid (standing). The hernia shown in **618** becomes obvious on standing.

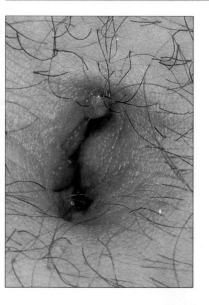

620 The discharging umbilicus.
This usually reflects poor hygiene and may be due to a patent urachus or the pouting granulation tissue of **a pilonidal sinus**.

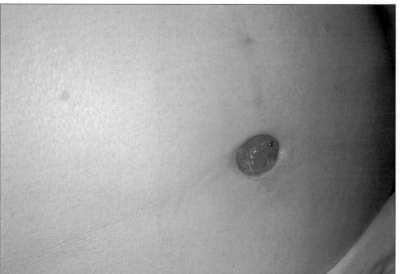

621 The umbilical secondary deposit. Abdominal primary tumours (stomach or colon) may seep through the umbilicus and appear as secondary nodules deep in the opening. They are often felt before they are seen.

ABDOMINAL FULLNESS

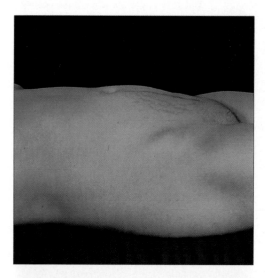

622 Abdominal proptosis—1. This is a frequent cause of transient abdominal swelling and feeling of distension that may then disappear without the passage of flatus. It may come on rapidly and the patient is obliged to wear loose clothes. It is a little recognised and rarely sought physical sign.

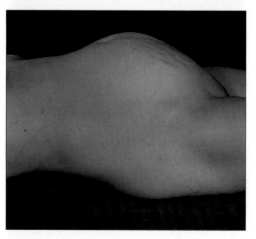

623 Abdominal proptosis—2.[117] "Now show me how it looks..."—the patient can often demonstrate the change in abdominal contour while being examined by a combination of diaphragmatic descent and increased lumbar lordosis. It is nearly always a manifestation of 'stress'. When chronic it is the mechanism of pseudocyesis.

---

[117]A delightful paper well repaying a trip to the library. Alvarez WC. Hysterical type non gaseous abdominal bloating. *Arch. Int. Med.*, 1949, **84**: 217–45.

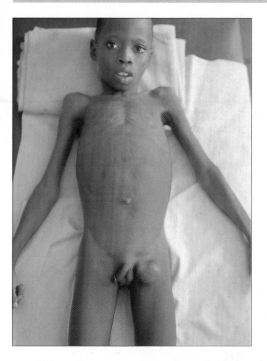

624 Abdominal fullness. This youth has umbilical eversion and distension with some dilated superficial abdominal veins. The swelling in the left groin lies below the inguinal ligament and must be differentiated from a lymph gland or aneurysm and a hernia, varix or pointing psoas abscess. The differentiating feature of the two groups is the presence of a cough impulse and reducibility. If this youth with abdominal **tuberculosis** has a tuberculous abscess that has extended from the iliac region, another swelling will be found above the ligament and fluctuation will be present between the two swellings. Then check the spine.

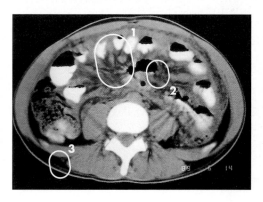

625 Tuberculosis peritonitis (computerised tomographic scan of the abdomen). This scan of the abdomen shows a characteristic thickening of the bowel wall and the mesentery, which can be seen fanning out from its root. The appearance is like that of wax running down the side of a candle (1). There is also 'spotty' infiltration (2) of mesenteric fat (compare it to the fat of the abdominal wall (3)). This appearance is very suggestive of lymphoma, but in this setting tuberculosis must always be considered.

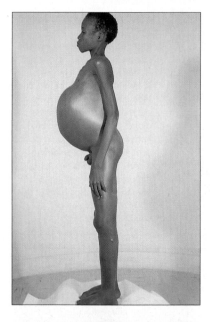

626 Gross ascites due to tuberculosis. An emaciated yet oedematous man with peripheral oedema and a tense fluid-filled belly. Look at the neck veins, and check for pulsus paradoxus to exclude constrictive pericarditis.

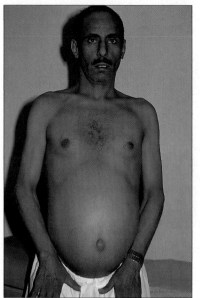

627 Ascites due to cirrhosis of the liver. The sclerae are yellow, the abdomen is distended and the umbilical hernia is full of fluid. Minor gynaecomastia is present. Other signs to look for include shiny nails, white nails, palmar erythema, scratch marks, spider naevi, oedema, Troisier's sign, the gall bladder, and venous distension.

DILATED VEINS ON THE TRUNK

Dilated veins on the trunk may be due to a vena caval block or compression, portal hypertension or portal vein thrombosis. The consequences may be varices, splenomegaly, dilated surface collateral veins or intractable haemorrhoids.

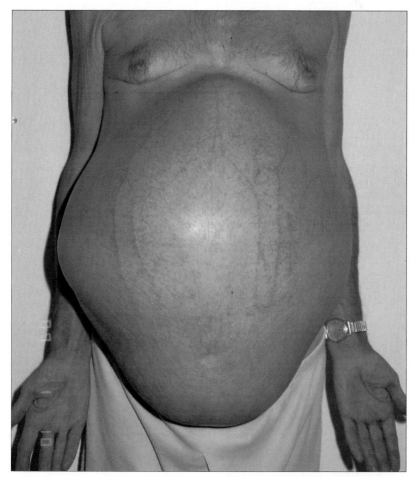

628 'Ascites' and dilated veins. A heavy drinker (40 units a day) with long-standing resistant ascites, palmar erythema and conspicuous abdominal veins. The direction of flow is shown in **629–31**.

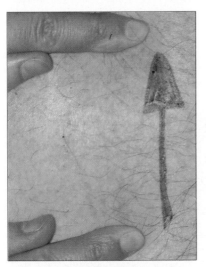

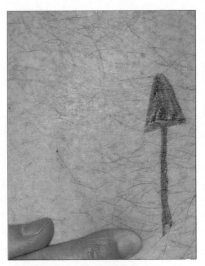

629 Veins and the direction of flow—1. The direction of flow of the veins shown in **628** can be determined by placing the opposed fingers together and separating them while pressing on the vein.

630 Veins and the direction of flow—2. When the upper finger is released the vein does not fill.

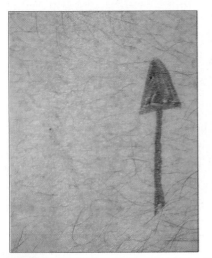

631 Veins and the direction of flow—3. On releasing the lower finger, the flow is upwards. This suggests inferior vena caval obstruction rather than collaterals in portal hypertension when blood from the left branch of the portal vein reaches the umbilicus via paraumbilical veins; the direction of flow is then away from the umbilicus. This man's ascites (*see* **628**) was in fact a large cyst of the appendix, which explained the curious profile of the abdomen.

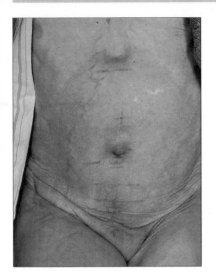

632 Para-aortic metastases. These lead to inferior vena caval compression and the formation of collateral venous channels.

Patient observation of the abdomen from the end of the bed with an oblique light, may show characteristic shadows.

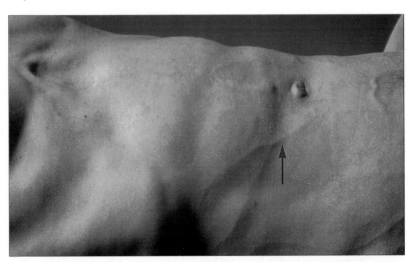

633 A big liver with secondary nodules. Carcinoma of the oesophagus and hepatic secondaries. An extensive venous collateral network can be seen in the lower abdomen bypassing the obstructed vena cava. The edge of a large liver (arrow) can be seen just above the umbilicus on either side of the midline.

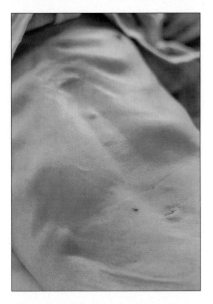

634 The scaphoid abdomen. This is the term given to the concavity of the abdomen found in dehydrating weight loss and sometimes with abdominal rigidity without respiratory excursion. There is a secondary deposit in the midline, which moves on breathing. An epigastic hernia through the linea alba looks the same, but does not move.

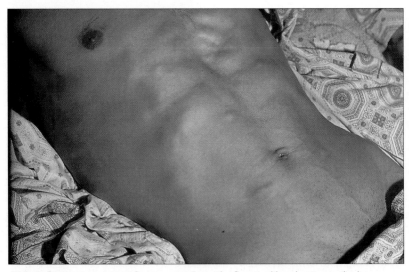

635 Inferior vena caval compression. The flow in dilated veins on the lower abdomen and lateral chest is upwards. There is a nodule in the liver, which moves with breathing, in the epigastrium.

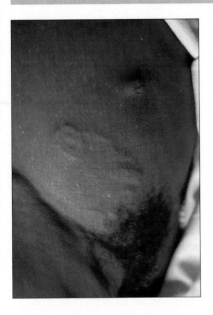

636 Ascites and the *serpent* under the skin. "A serpent do bite in my belly!" was this patient's description of his symptoms, unaware that indeed there was one, though no longer alive. The ascites and everted umbilicus are due to tuberculous disease and there is an outline of a dead subcutaneous guinea worm (*Dracunculus medinensis*).

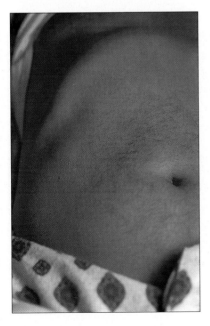

637 The visible gallbladder. This is moving with respiration and lying laterally. It is easy to see how faulty selection of a site for liver biopsy can be perilously close to it. If there is obstructive jaundice and a palpable gall bladder the obstruction is in the common bile duct. A stone in the cystic duct and another in the common bile duct is the exception.

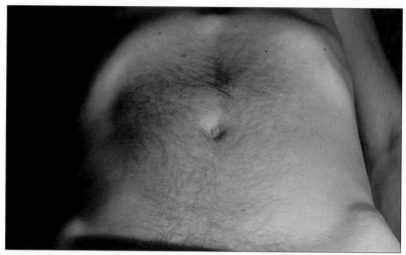

638 Visible peristalsis—1. The period of observation should not be too short or the visible peristalsis will be missed. A little patience can be rewarded by the sight of the wave rolling across under the abdominal wall. The obstructed colon is heaped up in the right upper quadrant.

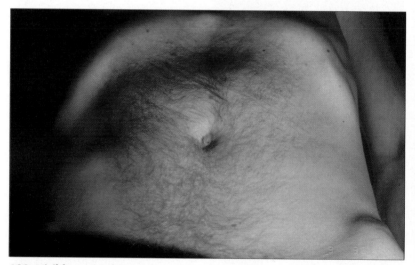

639 Visible peristalsis—2. Peristalsis moves across as a wave from right to left along the transverse colon and coincides with a colicky pain. This man has a colonic carcinoma.

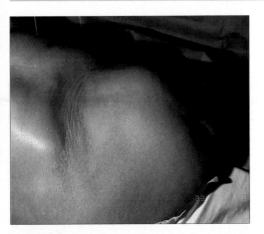

640 The swelling arising from the pelvis. A large pelvic swelling (his big bladder) is thrown into prominence by oblique light.

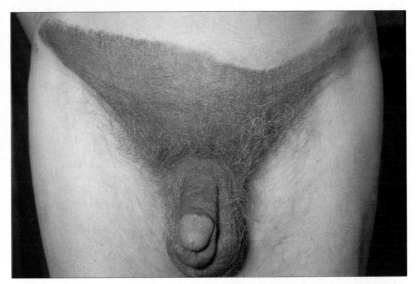

641 The perils of coughing. Bouts of coughing in a patient with bronchitis led to sudden abdominal pain. A shearing rupture of the epigastric artery in the rectus abdominis produces a mass in the upper abdomen if the superior epigastric artery is affected, and in the lower abdomen if the inferior epigastric artery is involved. The pain is worse on contraction of the abdominal muscles when the lump may disappear as it lies behind the muscle and mimics an intra-abdominal mass. The blood will track and is limited by the fascia. Cough complications include syncope, rib fracture, subconjunctival haemorrhage, cough headache, purpura, hernia and stress incontinence.

THE LOWER BACK

The lower back is often overlooked in the search for physical signs.

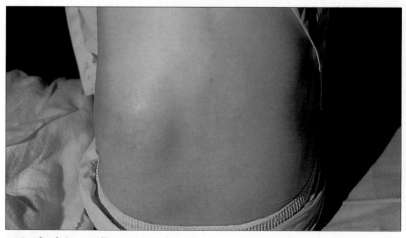

642 The loin swelling. This diabetic with ketoacidosis shows filling of the loin bulges with overlying erythema. This is due to a perinephric abscess presenting after a period of malaise and loin pain.

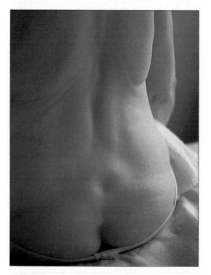

643 The sacral pad. When the back is examined check for pitting oedema over the sacrum—pressure should be firm and sustained. When patients are first seen in outpatients or the consulting room they have been mobile and upright. Once in bed, ankle oedema may disappear only to reappear, if looked for, over the sacrum.

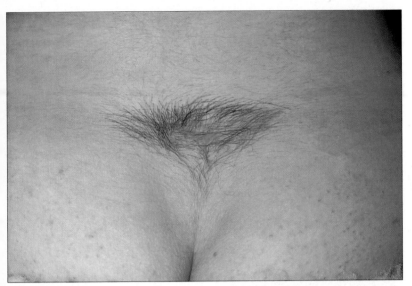

644 Spina bifida occulta. There is a tuft of hair and an area of atrophic skin overlying the sacrum at the apex of the natal cleft. Minor forms of spinal dysraphism may be associated with intraspinal abnormalities and neurological changes. If symptoms are present there may be external physical signs.

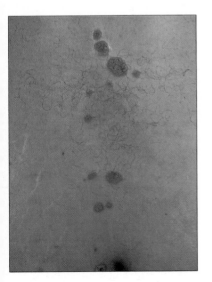

645 Sacral psoriasis. Psoriasis may be present over the sacrum. It may be the only place where it is active at the time that the patient is seen. Other sites include the penis, scalp, knees and elbows.

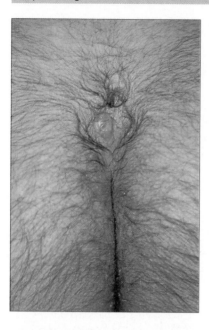

646 Pilonidal sinus. The pouting granulation tissue at the opening of the sinus in a hairy natal cleft is usually present.

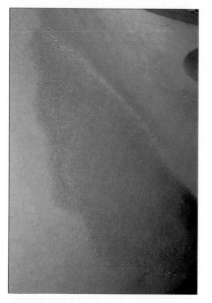

647 Groin itch. Fungal infection of the skin fold. The dry dermis is more resistant to infection, which may account for ringworm's predilection for sweaty toe clefts and skin folds. The appearance results from a combination of keratin destruction and inflammatory response. Some species have a predilection for a particular site—*Microsporum audouini* and tinea capitis, *Trichophyton rubrum* and tinea pedis. Both may cause tinea corporis.

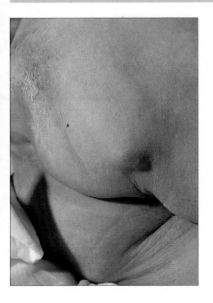

648 The rear view. Rheumatoid nodules on the ischial tuberosity are easily overlooked. Infection and ulceration of the nodule may lead to great discomfort.

THE PERINEUM AND ANUS—EASILY MISSED SIGNS!

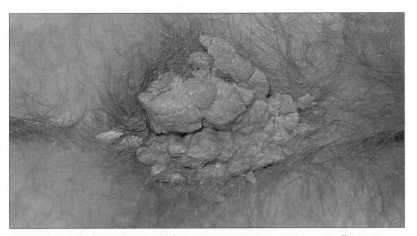

649 Anogenital warts—condylomata acuminatum. Human papilloma virus stimulates the production of basal cells in the dermis. These warts are common in sexually active adults and involve the genitalia and perineum. In the immunosuppressed they may be florid. On the cervix they are precancerous and they are associated with anal cancer in homosexuals.

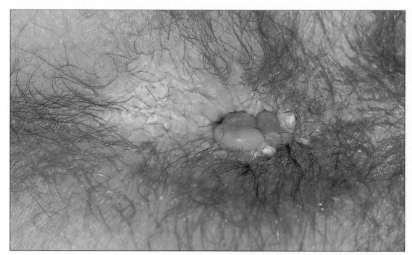

650 Pruritus ani. The lichenified pink-white skin change typical of chronic itch, and skin tags, the remnants of thrombosed external piles. The cause is usually long past and remains a cycle of itch–scratch–itch.

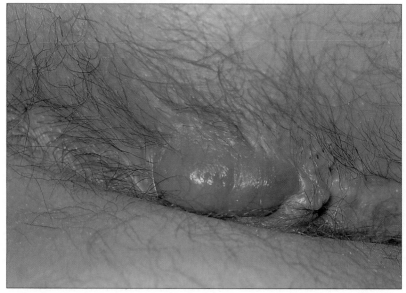

651 The thrombosed external haemorrhoid. A painful but self-limiting condition.

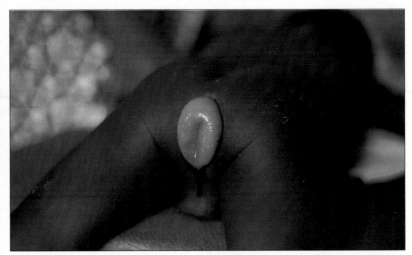

652 Prolapsed rectal mucosa. A common finding in severe diarrhoea, especially in children. Manual replacement may be all that is needed. In the UK may be seen in a normal toddler.

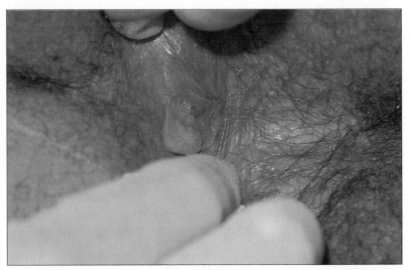

653 The anal fissure. An acute painful condition. Parting the skin folds will bring the apex into view even if digital examination is difficult. The sentinel pile is seen at the external edge, with the scarlet of the fissure deep to it.

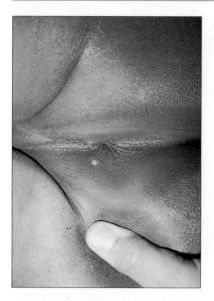

654 The anal fistula. Approximately 25% of patients with intestinal Crohn's disease have an anal lesion during their illness. It may be the presenting feature and antedate the abdominal disease. Biopsy is important to exclude tuberculosis.

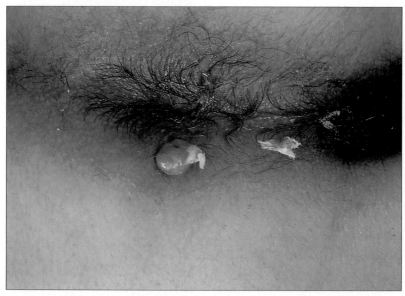

655 Anal fistula in Crohn's disease. The skin tags look succulent and soft, but have a very firm consistency; the dusky blue appearance is characteristic.

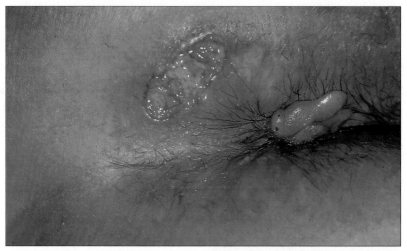

656 Anal tags and fistula in Crohn's disease. Many fistulae may be present and are often surprisingly painless.

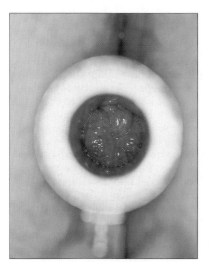

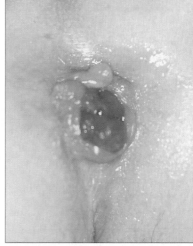

657 Internal haemorrhoids. As the patient strains the haemorrhoids fill the proctoscope. On withdrawal the haemorrhoids prolapse and are captured by the anal sphincter. These are a common cause of rectal bleeding and insidious anaemia, but should never be assumed to be the prime cause of rectal bleeding.

THE STOOLS

It pays to look at the stools. A patient's verbal description may not mean the same to the physician.

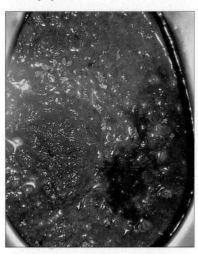

658 The purgative addict. Self-induced diarrhoea—remember that patients may be economical with the truth! This self-induced diarrhoea revealed by the addition of caustic soda to the stool, turning it red, was due to **surreptitious phenolphthalein ingestion**.

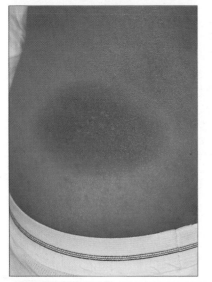

659 A fixed drug eruption (and phenolphthalein ingestion). The characteristic of this eruption is that the rash recurs at the same site on each exposure to the drug. Many drugs are implicated: tetracycline, sulphonamides, aspirin, paracetamol, phenolphthalein and benzodiazepines. The rash commonly occurs on the limbs. This patient had an eruption whenever he took laxatives containing phenolphthalein. The post-inflammatory pigmentation may persist indefinitely.

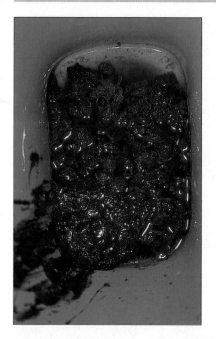

660 Beetroot and panic![118] A

change in stool colour causes alarm. It may mimic rectal bleeding. A more mundane explanation may be food ingestion. Beeturia is the excretion of red beetroot pigment (betalaine) in urine and faeces, an experience shared by 14% of people. It results from colonic absorption of the pigment and is more frequent in untreated iron deficiency and achlorhydira. The pigment is decolourised in non-beeturic individuals by non-enzymatic action in the stomach and colon. Whether or not an individual has beeturia seems to be determined by the colon and will occur into an ileostomy. The red colour is decolourised by gastric acid and by colonic bacteria but preserved by oxalic acid if present in foods such as rhubarb and spinach, rich in oxalic acid.

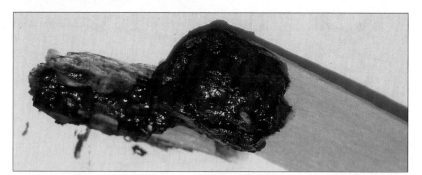

661 The melaena stool. A non-insulin-dependent diabetic began to sweat profusely and felt dizzy. His doctor daughter measured his blood sugar and gave oral glucose. Sweating persisted. He became hypotensive. Rectal examination disclosed the classical melaena stool of dark black-red colour produced by partly digested blood from a bleeding peptic ulcer. This was secondary to oral non-steroidal anti-inflammatory drugs for an arthritic knee. Oral iron may produce a grey stool and be confused with altered blood.

[118]Eastwood M, Nyhlin H. Beeturia and colonic oxalic acid. *Quart. J. Med.*, 1995, **88**, 711–17.

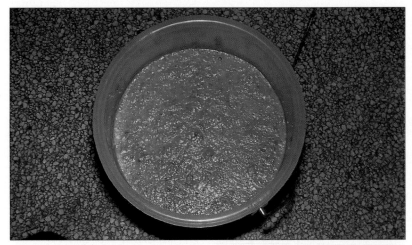

662 The bowl of steatorrhoea. A formed stool does not exclude steatorrhoea, but the fat-laden stool is usually offensive, bulky, floats, and is difficult to flush away. A normal stool may also float if it has a high gas content.

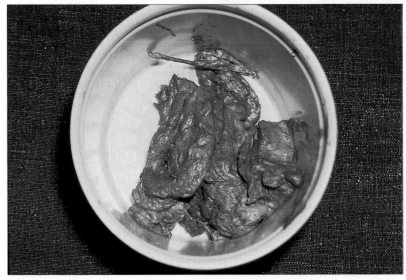

663 The silver stool. This appearance is produced by steatorrhoea and mild blood loss, in this case due to a carcinoma of the duodenal ampulla.

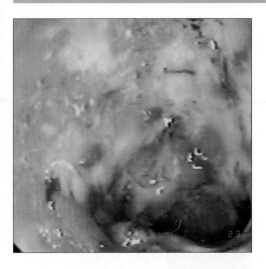

664 Pseudomembrane.
Antibiotic-associated colitis leads to sloughing of the colonic mucosa. Although the single most important factor is associated antibiotic use this condition was first described in the nineteenth century and may complicate serious medical illness. The onset may be insidious or catastrophic, and a high index of suspicion is essential. The membrane may be seen in the lumen at endoscopy.

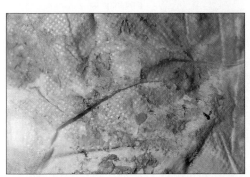

665 Pseudomembrane in the stool. The membrane is also seen in the stool.

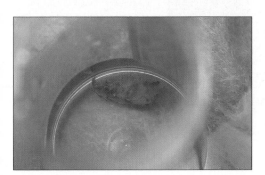

666 Pseudomembrane slough *in situ*. The slough appears as a sheet if suspended in saline.

COLOUR CHANGES IN THE URINE

The colour may be:
- White if there is a large volume or an osmotic diuresis.
- Yellow/orange if it is concentrated.
- Yellow/orange if it contains bile.
- Orange if on rifampicin.
- Red if there is haemoglobinuria.
- Red/pink if there is beeturia.
- Yellow going grey on standing, in alkaptonuria.
- Darkening to port wine colour on standing, in porphyria.
- Red if there is phenolphthalein, in alkaline urine.
- Black if there is melanuria.
- Black if there is methaemoglobinuria.
- Green/blue if it contains methylene blue.

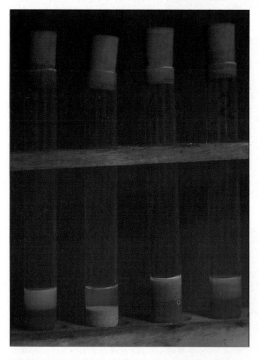

667 The urine in porphyria. A young girl, with abdominal pain and distress had repeated admissions over a six-month period in the same north London area. She died on the eve of the publication of the BMJ article by Ida Macalpine and Richard Hunter on the illness of George III[119]. The next morning one of the medical team read the article and aspirated urine from the bladder post-mortem. The diagnosis missed in life! The urine darkens on standing (the port wine change) and fluoresces in ultraviolet light. On the left is a control and the patient's urine and on the right the patient's stool and a control.

[119]MacAlpine I. Hunter. The "insanity" of King George III: a classic Case of Porphyria. *BMJ*. Jan. 8, 1966. **5479**, 65–71.

THE PENIS

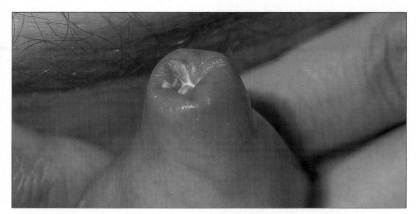

668 Balanitis (*Candidiasis*). A diabetic's sugary urine leads to balanitis and *Candidiasis* infection, the inflammation leading to phimosis. Trauma, chemical irritants and contact dermatitis from condoms may all present as balanitis.

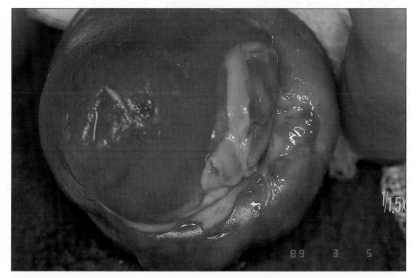

669 Erosive balanitis. In diabetics anaerobic infection may lead to tissue destruction. A primary syphilitic chancre must be excluded, but balanitis may be gonococcal.

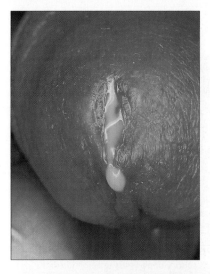

670 The urethral discharge. The urethritis often leads to a creamy purulent discharge. The appearance is variable. A clear discharge may be normal. Pathological causes include gonorrhoea, chlamydia, *Ureaplasma*, *Trichomonas*, herpes, *Candida* or a foreign body. Microscopic examination is essential.

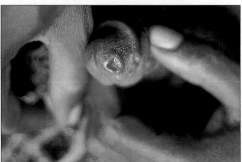

671 A lesion on the glans penis. This may be acute or longstanding. Primary syphilis leads to a painless ulcer with a firm base like a small button and inguinal gland enlargement.

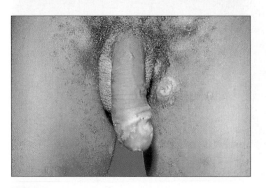

672 Condylomata (secondary syphilis) in the groin. Later papules in moist areas may enlarge into flat moist infectious condylomata.

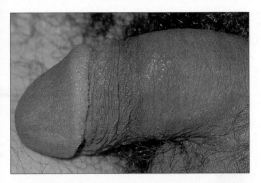

673 Genital herpes vesicle. A more common problem is genital ulceration due to herpes infection. This is recurrent and there is usually a story of vesicle production.

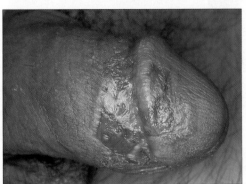

674 Genital herpes — confluent broken vesicles. By the time of presentation the vesicles have usually ruptured, producing a non-specific confluent ulcerated area.

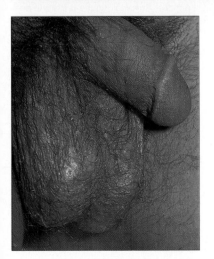

675 Herpes on the scrotum. Herpes may occur anywhere on the genitals.

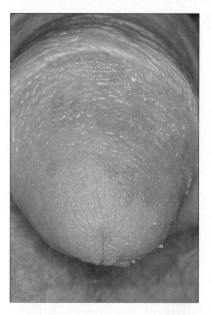

676 Psoriasis of the glans. Some chronic skin diseases also have a predilection for the glans. **Psoriasis** may look slightly different (white and moist) on the uncircumcised glans.

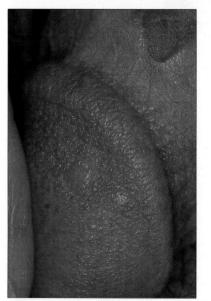

677 Lichen planus of the glans. Alhough more usually seen on the wrists and ankles, lichen planus may be seen on the glans. A typical plaque is present and an annular lesion on the shaft.

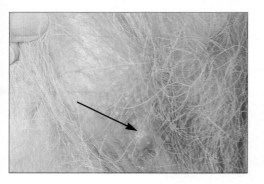

678 Feel the testes!
Examination of the rectum and genitalia are two areas where attention to clinical method may pay dividends. This patient came to England to consult doctors for a 'general check-up'. At the end of the negative abdominal examination, the scrotum was examined and a swelling with a sinus was found. On remonstrating with the patient he said that this was his reason for travelling to England. He had waited for a doctor to find it. The patient's method of quality control!

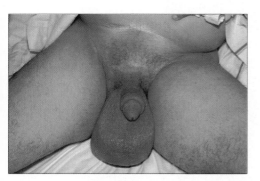

679 Scrotal oedema due to carcinoma of the rectum. The lax skin predisposes to oedema localisation. Usually associated with hypoalbuminaemia or cardiac failure, it can be due to regional lymphatic obstruction.

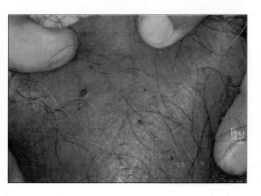

680 Cherry angiomas (*syn.* Campbell de Morgan spots). These are common with increasing age. Histologically they are angiokeratomas. They may vary in number and may disappear. Similar spots may occur on the trunk.

THE LOWER LIMB

The lower limb is usually covered by trousers, tights or hosiery and only seen on demand unless part of the presenting complaint.

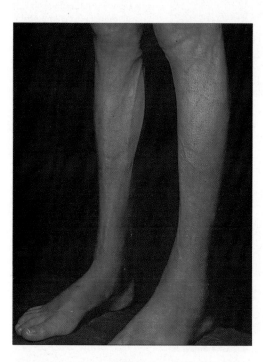

681 The thin leg of anorexia nervosa. This shows emaciation and brown pigmentation. The skin is dry and scaly, like the craquelure of an oil painting, and this is a feature of malnutrition. Oedema is unusual and is due less to hypoproteinaemia than to a relative maintenance of the extracellular fluid compared to loss of body mass (see **142**).

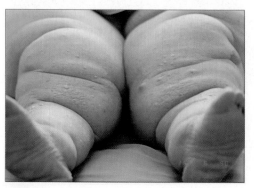

682 The fat leg of obesity. This may be complicated by oedema, a result of pressure from the abdominal apron and folds of limb fat on venous and lymphatic channels. This weight further increases mean capillary pressure and potential for oedema, already aggravated by reduced lymphatic and venous flow from reduced calf pump action due to a lack of movement.

Determine the cause of pitting oedema. If it is confined to one limb it is likely to be due to venous or lymphatic obstruction.

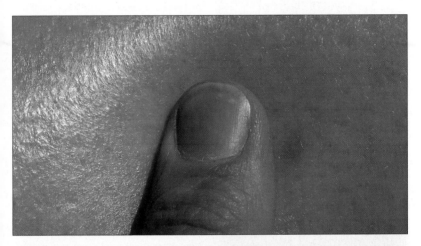

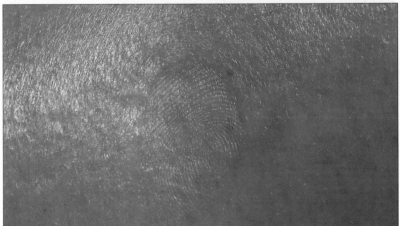

683, 684 Pitting oedema. This is the physical sign that the extravascular interstitial proportion of the extracellular fluid is increased. It is elicited by pressure for about 30 seconds. When the finger is removed a depression remains, which gradually fills in. In hypoproteinaemia, oedema may be generalised and is likely to be evident in the lax tissues of the face and be obvious on rising in the morning. In contrast the oedema of heart failure tends to collect in the legs at the end of the day and if bedbound will gravitate to the sacral area.

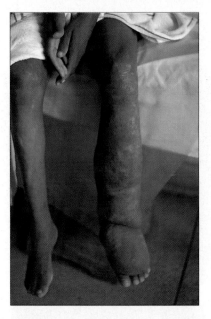

685 Lymphoedema due to filariasis. Blockage of the lymphatics by adult filarial parasites where they reproduce sexually to yield large numbers of microfilariae may lead to thick and brawny swelling. Non-filarial elephantiasis—podoconiosis[120]—is a disease of barefoot people that begins in the teens with an area of erythema and burning followed by persistent distal swelling of the foot and intermittent acute flares of discomfort. It is caused by penetration of the dermis by silica or aluminosilicates, which lead to lymphatic obstruction, and prevented by wearing shoes.

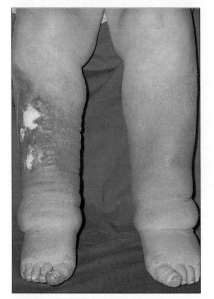

686 Congenital or Milroy's lymphoedema.[121] Inadequate lymph vessels lead to chronic oedema with fibrosis complicated by cellulitis and ulceration. The tissues are thickened and verrucous.

When lymphoedema is bilateral, cardiac, hepatic, renal or nutritional causes must be excluded by examination. Immobility—sitting up all night in a chair—is an important cause. Always check venous pressure and test the urine.

[120]Price EW. *Podoconiosis—non-filarial Elephantiasis.* Oxford University Press, 1990.
[121]William Forsyth Milroy, 1855–1942. An undescribed variety of hereditary oedema. *N. Y. Med. J.*, 1892, **56**: 505–8.

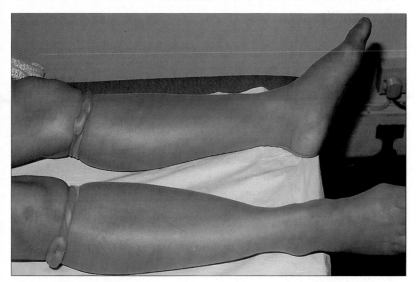

687 Oedema and garters. A complaint of oedema may have a prosaic cause. External compression of veins and lymphatics will lead to swelling.

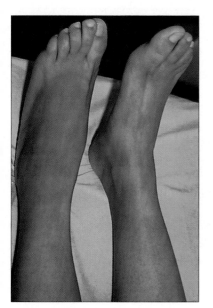

688 Pelvic tumours and oedema. A Cypriot seamstress complained of a swollen left leg. She operated a treadle sewing machine with her right foot for six days a week. No signs were found in the legs. The inexperienced physician explained that the inactive left leg did nor use the calf pump to increase lymph and venous flow and therefore this was sedentary unilateral oedema! He was embarrassed to find a large calcified pelvic fibroid on radiography which was easily felt when a full examination of the patient that included pelvic assessment was performed.

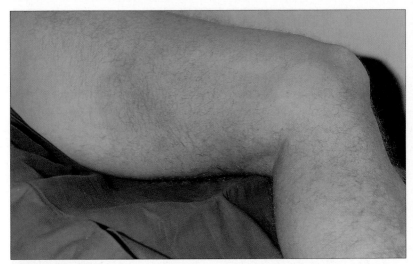

689 Acute superficial thrombophlebitis. There is a tender palpable vein with surrounding erythema, warmth and oedema. It gradually subsided over seven days.

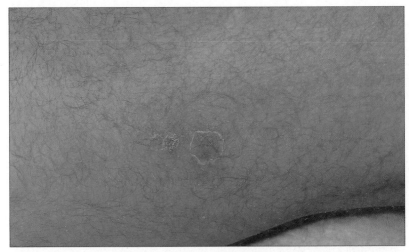

690 Resolving superficial thrombophlebitis. The overlying skin of the acute superficial thrombophlebitis shown in **689** peeled after the inflammation subsided. This condition is not associated with a risk of embolus. Migrating superficial thrombophlebitis may be a marker of an underlying malignancy.

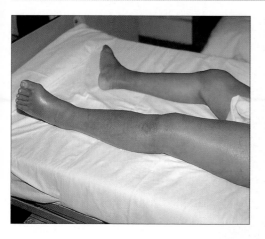

691 Deep venous thrombosis (DVT). There is extensive oedema in a leg with a proximal deep vein thrombosis and calf and thigh tenderness. Stasis, vascular damage and hypercoagulability are factors common to conditions in which venous thrombosis occurs (e.g. bedrest, surgery, trauma, malignant disease and hereditary and oestrogen-induced thrombophilic states). There may be no signs and tenderness if present may reflect the size of the inflammatory reaction.

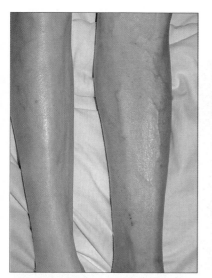

692 The residua of deep venous thrombosis (DVT). Following a DVT, recanalisation may occur, but residual obstruction in the deep venous system may lead to prominent superficial veins.

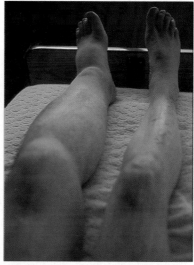

693 Residua of deep venous thrombosis—the chronic swollen leg. When the venous system is extensively blocked, severe residual swelling remains because the lymphatic channel cannot cope. This leads to chronic oedema.

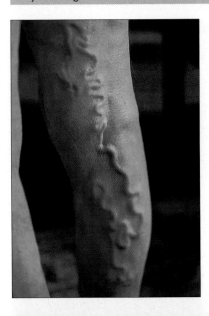

694 Varicose veins. These are superficial, dilated and tortuous. They are a complication of incompetent valves. As a result the head of pressure is transmitted to the unsupported vein and capillary.

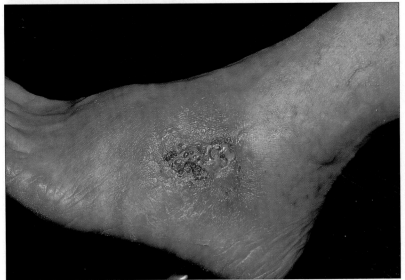

695 Varicose eczema. Irritating varicose eczema and hyperpigmentation related to leakage and breakdown of red cells may develop, followed by ulceration.

ERYSIPELAS

Erysipelas or St Anthony's fire is found on the face or limbs.

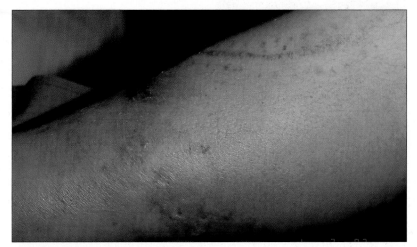

696 Erysipelas of the thigh (*see* 249). Infection with *Streptococcus pyogenes* to produce a cellulitis of the skin may be preceded by a systemic upset followed by erythema.

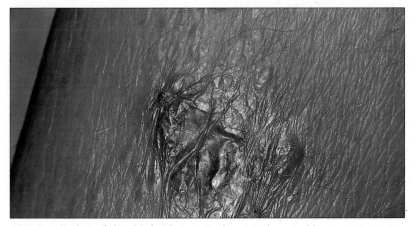

697 Erysipelas of the thigh (close-up). There may be overt blistering.

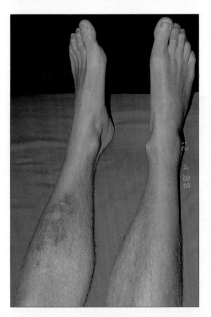

698 Erysipelas of the lower leg.
The physician patient diagnosed the red patch overlying the middle third of the tibia initially as flu due to the rigor, then as a groin hernia and then as an inguinal gland, and finally when the red hot tender area appeared on the leg, as erythema nodosum!

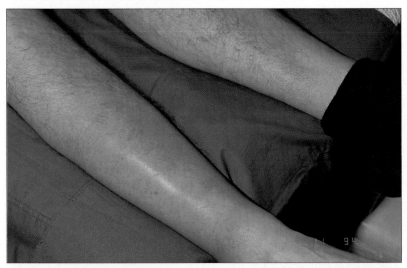

699 Erysipelas of the lower leg. Sudden rigors are followed 12 hours later by inflammation, which may spread.

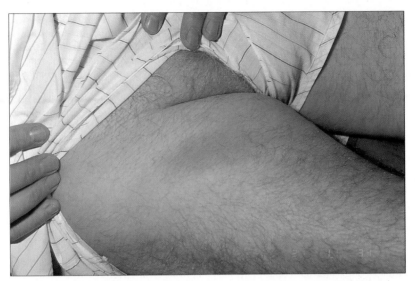

700 Erysipelas of the lower leg. It may spread up the leg and produce the red line of lymphangiitis.

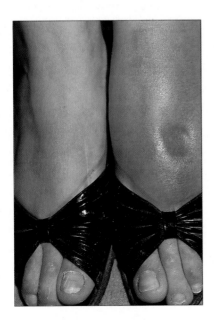

701 Erysipelas of the foot. A horse stable manager presented with rigors followed by groin soreness and only later noted redness and tenderness on the foot. The redness spread over the dorsum and the groin became more tender. Rapid improvement came with penicillin, but not before a doctor attempted treatment with a corticosteroid cream thinking the cause to be an allergy to leather.

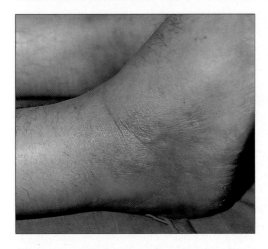

702 Stemmer's sign—the tethered subcutaneous tissue. Recurrent attacks of erysipelas may lead to firm oedema with tethering of the skin as a result of chronic fibrosis activated by the protein in the tissues and the decreased lymph flow. The skin over the toes and lower leg has become thickened and verrucous and a fold of skin cannot be easily pinched up, which is a characteristic of a lymphostatic[122] disorder typified by excess protein, oedema, chronic inflammation and excess fibrosis.

Operations on the hip, injections of adrenaline into the buttock, trauma, colonic surgery and lower limb operations may all produce the essentials of anoxic tissue and contamination with the spores of *Clostridium perfringens*.

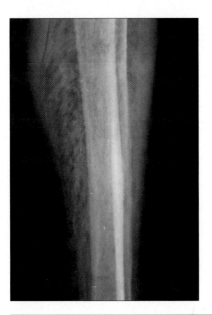

703 Gas gangrene. This man had auricular fibrillation and sustained a saddle embolus. A herbalist excoriated the skin and rubbed in a mixture of herbs and cow dung (*Clostridium perfringens* is found in animal or human faeces and in anoxic tissue). He presented 36 hours later with severe pain and toxicity. Prompt recognition is life saving. On the radiograph the gas in the tissues outlines the muscular septa and appears black against the white of the soft tissues, but may not be seen. It produces a subcutaneous crepitation to the touch and very severe toxicity in an alert patient.

---

[122]Mortimer P, Regnard C. Lymphostatic disorders. *Br. Med. J.*, 1986, **293**: 347–9.

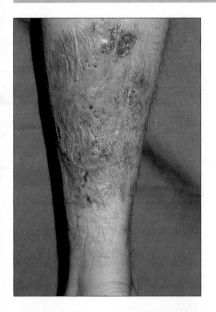

704 The Greek tanker captain with a weeping leg ulcer—1. This man had a six-month history of a discharging leg ulcer. He had had multiple courses of antibiotics, but no specific organism had been identified. On direct questioning he gave a story of bloody diarrhoea 10 years earlier. At colonoscopy burnt out colitis and stricture formation was seen. The gut histology showed Crohn's disease. This is **pyoderma gangrenosum**, which may complicate inflammatory bowel disease (Crohn's disease and ulcerative colitis), collagen disease (rheumatoid arthritis, systemic lupus erythematosus, Wegener's granulomatosis) and reticuloendothelial disorders (leukaemia and myeloma) (*see* **845–8**).

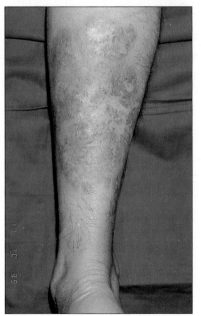

705 The Greek tanker captain with a weeping leg ulcer—2. After six weeks of oral prednisolone, his pyoderma gangrenosum had healed completely.

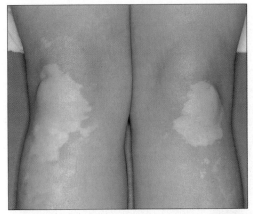

706 The knee—vitiligo (*see* 25). Destruction of melanocytes leads to total depigmentation of skin (vitiligo), which is a marker of autoimmune disease. It is often symmetrical and may be seen in association with Addison's disease (adrenocortical insufficiency), diabetes mellitus, pernicious anaemia and thyroid disease. However, test sensation to exclude leprosy and consider pityriasis.

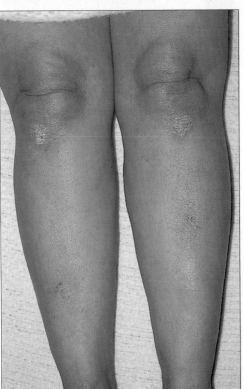

707 The knee—a religious Russian lady. Knee calluses may be due to trauma from kneeling when the weight is born by the tibial tubercles.

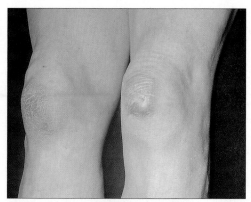

708 The knee—a housemaid's. Stretching forwards to scrub the floor or fit carpets may lead to soreness and swelling over the patella. This may lead to prepatellar or infrapatellar bursitis (*see* **709**).

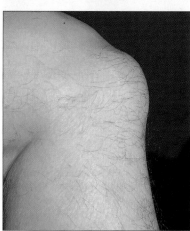

709 The knee—infrapatellar bursitis—the clergyman. Kneeling leads to bursitis which may affect clergymen and coal miners.

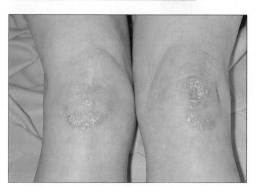

710 The knee—psoriasis. An important differential diagnosis.of infrapatellar bursitis is psoriasis of the knee. The silvery scale on the red base mimics the effect of friction (*see* **707**) and has a predilection for this site.

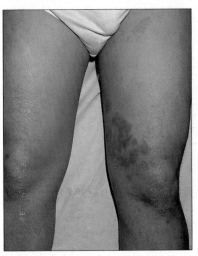

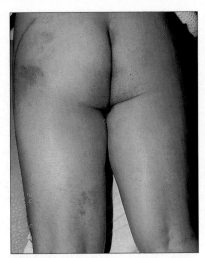

711 Herpes zoster (L3 dermatome).
Pain in the knee may be due to local joint disease or be referred from the hip joint. The pain of herpes zoster may add confusion if the anatomical distribution of the rash (L3) is not appreciated over the lower thigh and knee.

712 Herpes zoster L3 dermatome and extending to the buttock (see 711). Affecting part of the lateral buttock (*see diagram in appendix*).

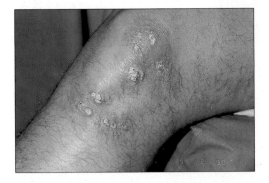

713 Cutaneous leishmaniasis at the knee. This resident of Riyadh, Saudi Arabia, spent a weekend in a rural oasis and his legs were bitten by sandflies. Three weeks later a red furuncle-like nodule developed. This ulcerated and was associated with satellite nodules in adjacent lymphatics. Infection is by a protozoan *Leishmania tropica, aethiopica* and *major* (Old World parasites), and *L. mexicana* and *brasiliensis* (New World ones). Transmitted by the bite of sandflies and prevalent on the borders of the Mediterranean, Arabia and central America.

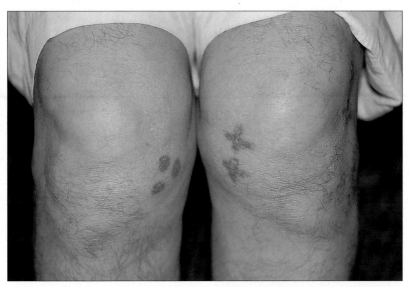

714 The site of pain of osteoarthritis of the knee. This is the sign of previous knee pain, which has been treated with counter-irritation and tattooing.

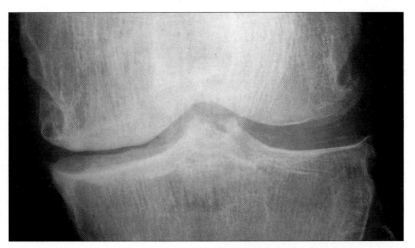

715 Osteoarthritis and chondrocalcinosis (radiograph of the knee). Since the pain of the osteoarthritic knee may be intermittent, ineffective treatment may appear to be effective. Calcification in the cartilage may be due to degenerative joint disease, but the differential diagnosis should be reviewed (*see* **466**).

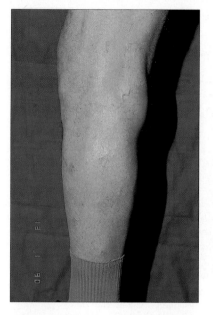

716a A popliteal cyst. This man turned around while out shopping thinking he had been struck from behind. Sudden pain behind the knee is due to rupture of a popliteal or Baker's cyst.[123] The cyst is an extension of the joint cavity, and the synovium may act as a ball valve pumping up the cyst. Sudden movement may increase the pressure and produce rupture leading to pain, and swelling down the back of the leg. It is usually associated with rheumatoid or degenerative joint disease. The differential diagnosis includes acute deep vein thrombosis (which must be differentiated because anticoagulation may lead to bleeding into the tissues) and ruptured plantaris or medial head of gastrocnemius. In the presence of any acute arthritis of the knee it is more probable that rupture has occurred.

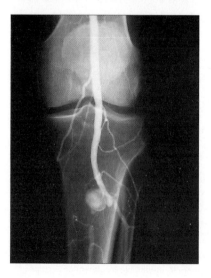

716b Mycotic aneurysm. A leaking popliteal aneurysm may cause pain in the popliteal fossa. This man with bacterial endocarditis complained of aching pain behind the knee for two weeks before the aneurysm was appreciated.

---

[123]William Morrant Baker, 1839–96, described in 1885.

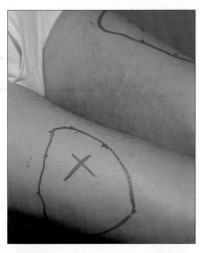

717 The thigh with dysaesthesiae.
Pain from L2–4 root compression may be confused with the entrapment neuropathy of the lateral femoral cutaneous nerve (**meralgia paraesthetica**). The lateral femoral cutaneous nerve arises from L2–3 sensory roots, enters the thigh under the lateral edge of the inguinal ligament just medial to the anterior superior iliac spine, and supplies the anterior lateral thigh. It may be compressed by belts or tightly laced corsets. Meralgia paraesthetica is common in obesity, pregnancy and after coronary artery bypass surgery. The burning pain and area of abnormal sensation may be mapped out with a sharp instrument. It is often bilateral.

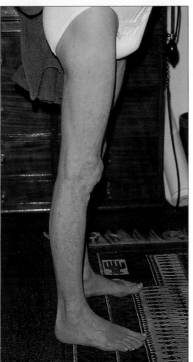

718 Diabetic amyotrophic wasting of the thigh. This diabetic has severe pain in the legs and recent muscle weakness, which is particularly noticeable on climbing stairs. There is wasting of the right upper thigh. Contrast this with the full left quadriceps. Diabetic amyotrophy is a multifocal neuropathy. It is an asymmetrical motor syndrome affecting the anterior thigh muscles and producing wasting of acute onset. This is often accompanied with pain, which is worse at night. There may be little sensory loss. Other diabetic neuropathies are: symmetrical sensory polyneuropathy, which may affect the cranial nerves—the oculomotor (iii) nerve sparing pupillary enervation and the facial (vii) nerve. Other entrapment neuropathies are also more common in diabetics.

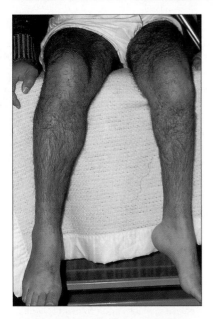

719 Quadriceps wasting. Muscle wasting is a common sign of disuse. It occurs rapidly with bedrest of even a short duration and will be symmetrical, and after injury or lower motor neurone denervation, as in **poliomyelitis**. Upper motor neurone lesions by comparison produce little wasting. Here a lower motor neurone lesion in childhood led to growth impairment and a disparity in leg length.

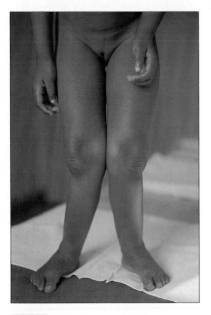

720 Rickets. Varus and valgus deformity or a combination of the two (windswept legs) may result from the mechanical stresses on the soft unmineralised osteoid.

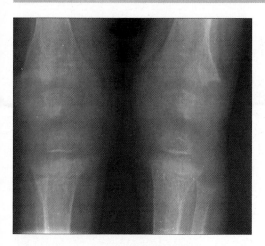

721 Florid rickets (radiograph). This shows the expanded epiphyseal plate of vitamin D deficiency (rickets).

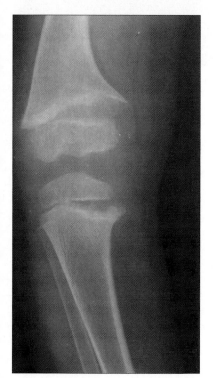

722 Healing rickets (radiograph). Calcification occurs at the epiphyseal plate, but the soft osteoid has deformed producing a bow leg deformity.

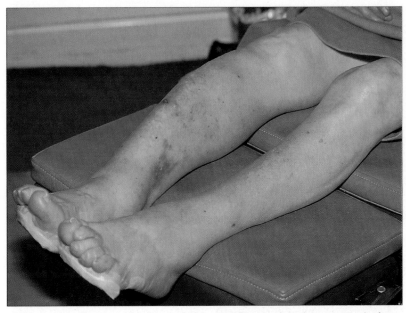

723 Paget's disease—the bowed tibia. An elderly lady with increasing deafness and an aching, bowed, warm and expanded right tibia (*see* **106, 107**).

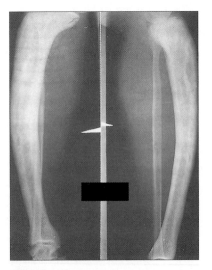

724 Pagetic tibia (radiograph). Radiologically the dense expanded pagetic bone contrasts with the normal fibula.

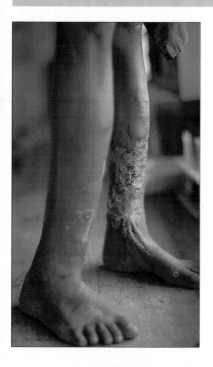

725 Sabre tibia in yaws. In the deformity produced by a spirochaete, the sabre-like deformity is secondary to a periostitis.

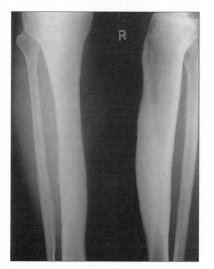

726 Sabre tibia in yaws (radiograph). Periostitis leads to thickening. The leg itself remains straight because the thickening is on the anterior surface of the bone. A similar appearance may occur in the periostitis of syphilis and should not be confused with the pagetic deformity.

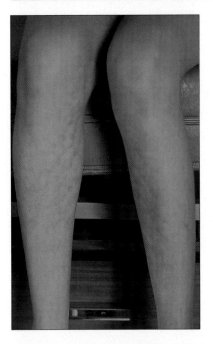

727 The woman who felt the cold—erythema ab igne. This reticular pigmentation and telangiectasia, usually on the legs, results from chronic and repeated exposure to radiant (infrared) heat. It can occur with other heat sources (*see* **613**). Once common in the United Kingdom when huddling around a source of radiant heat was the way to keep warm, it may still be seen if an open fire is available. This person sits in front of the fire because both medial aspects are affected. The side on which the individual usually sits can often be determined from the pattern affecting the lateral aspect of one leg and the medial aspect of the other. Hypothyroidism and hypothermia must be excluded. Erythema ab igne should be differentiated from livedo reticularis (*see* **728**).

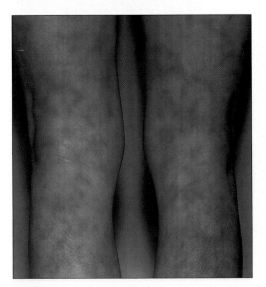

728 Livedo reticularis. In livedo reticularis the change is symmetrical and there is telangiectasia alone without pigmentation. The change is a 'net-like' pattern of cyanotic change, which increases in the cold. It is related to the cones of skin supplied by an individual arteriole, with cyanosis appearing at the edge of each cone base. It is caused by abnormalities of the arteriole. Secondary livedo may be related to an arteritis such as that of polyarteritis nodosa and cryoglobulinaemia.

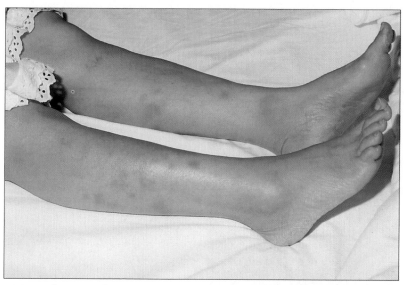

729 Erythema nodosum. Arthralgia and a tender rash developed during the course of a mycoplasma pneumonia. The frequent appearance on the front of the shin may be related to poor clearance of antigen from this site of slow lymphatic drainage.

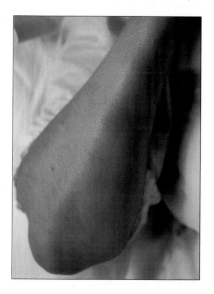

730 Erythema nodosum on the ulnar (nodose). These tender red swellings are usually seen on the shins or the arms.

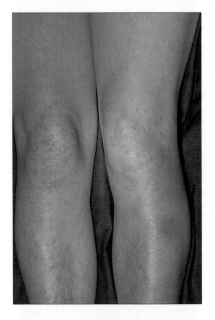

731 Erythema nodosum of the leg. Bruising is a feature. There is injury to small blood vessels in the dermis and subcutaneous tissue leading to a vasculitic panniculitis with tenderness, erythema and nodularity. Arthralgia may be seen. It may last from 2–10 weeks or more. It is a reaction pattern to drugs or infection and may be associated with a streptococcal sore throat, tuberculosis, sarcoidoisis, neoplasia, the contraceptive pill and pregnancy. It may be seen with chronic inflammatory bowel diseases, but is commonest after viral infections. A chest radiograph is a valuable investigation.

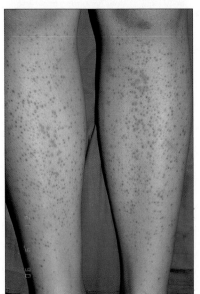

732 Cutaneous vasculitis— Henoch-Schönlein purpura. In cutaneous vasculitis (a response by small blood vessels to injury) there is nearly always non-thrombocytopenic purpura, along with some urticarial lesions and slight bruising as fading takes place. It has a predilection for the lower leg and shin, perhaps due to poor anatomical facilities for clearing antigen or complexes (*see* **383**).

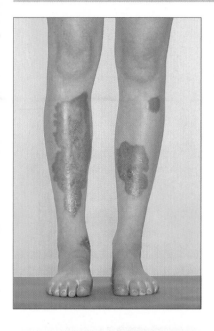

733a Necrobiosis lipoidica. The histological change of a palisading granuloma leads to a chronic area of fibrosis, which may persist and scar in necrobiosis lipoidica. This is commonly seen on the legs and may occur alone or in association with diabetes mellitus or acquired immune deficiency syndrome (AIDS).

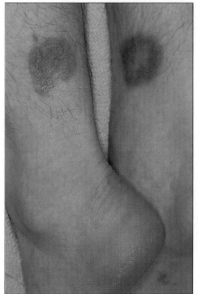

733b Necrobiosis lipoidica (close-up). The lesion is red-gold and has a slightly raised edge and an atrophic centre.

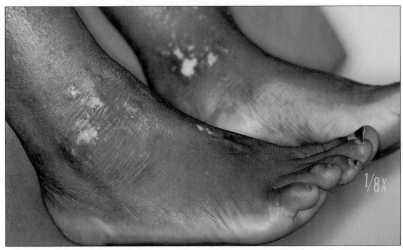

734 Itchy ankles. An irritating rash at the ankles and wrists with violaceous flat-topped shiny plaques. This is a typical site of lower limb **lichen planus**.

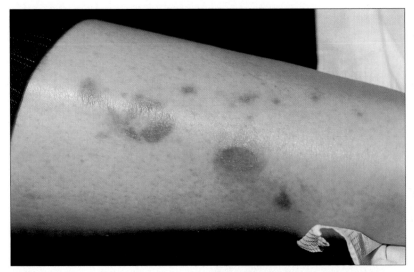

735 Diabetic dermopathy. This is characterised by trivial pigmented macules on the shins, which may begin as dull red papules, and may blister and become scaly leaving a depressed scar.

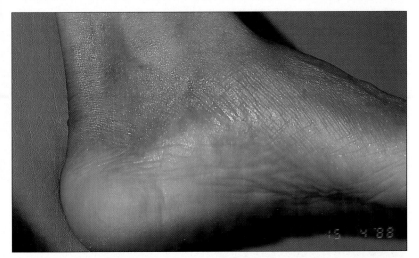

736 Sweaty feet (hyperhidrosis). Although sweaty feet are often the prerogative of youth they may reflect disease. Usually common and normal, but uncommonly abnormal—the sweating may be exertional or due to emotion, climate, fever, hypoglycaemia, acromegaly or thyrotoxicosis.

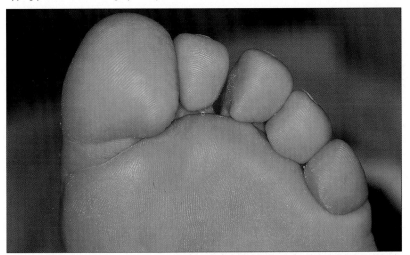

737 Sweaty feet—excess soft tissue (acromegaly)! This sweaty foot is shoe-moulded, but there is also an excess of soft tissue spreading into the interdigital clefts from the pulp of the toes and the sole of the foot. An acromegalic's feet may increase in size.

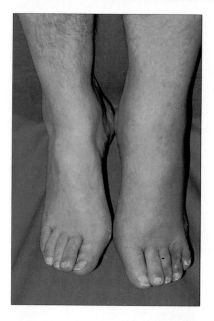

738 Reflex sympathetic dystrophy—algodystrophy. This patient had had a swollen, painful and discoloured left foot for six months and had no history of preceding trauma. The upper or lower limb may be involved and usually there is a history of previous trauma, hemiparesis, myocardial infarction or fracture. Local pain swelling and trophic skin change are followed by demineralisation of bone (see **739**).

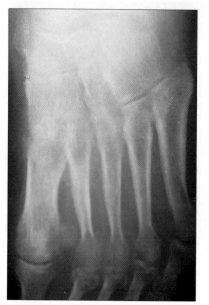

739 Reflex sympathetic dystrophy (radiograph). The radiograph of the left foot (**739**) shows demineralisation affecting the bones of the forefoot.

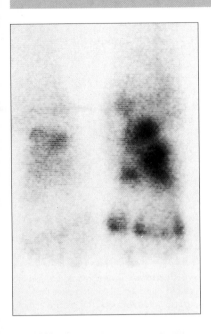

740 Reflex sympathetic dystrophy (bone scan). Demineralisation, as seen on the radiograph (*see* **739**), may be preceded by a positive change on the radioisotope scan. This is essentially a disturbance of the autonomic nervous system, but the exact mechanism remains unclear.

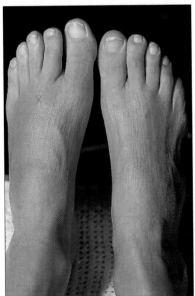

741 Pain in the forefoot. After two weeks of tourism around Europe this patient complained of pain in the forefoot. The 'X' marks the site of maximum pain. The initial radiograph showed nothing, but a further radiograph a month later confirmed the diagnosis of a **stress or march fracture**. The tibia, distal fibula and second and third metatarsals are the commonest sites.

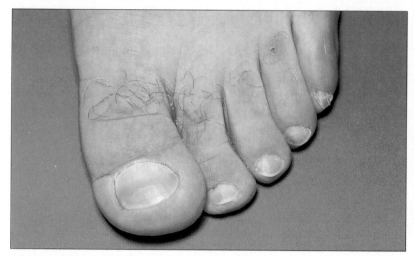

742 Pretibial myxoedema for nearly two decades. Severe thyrotoxicosis with malignant exophthalmos was complicated by a raised pink skin thickening over the dorsum of the feet and over the shin. Finger nail clubbing developed. The picture is that of thyroid acropachyderma or acropachy.

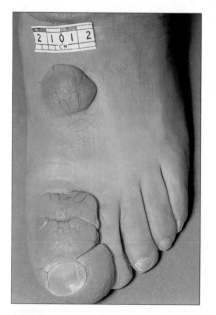

743 Pretibial myxoedema 1972. The thickening progressed to produce a typical appearance.

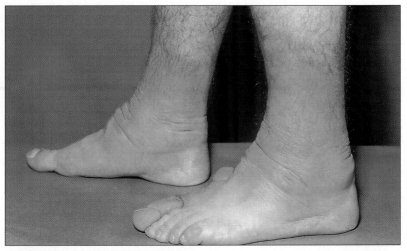

744 Pretibial myxoedema 1974. This shows the typical appearance over the lower leg.

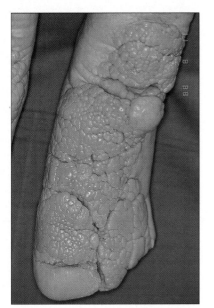

745 Pretibial myxoedema 1988.
Ultimately a lymphoedema-like state developed. Ophthalmopathy and the dermopathy are both characterised by an accumulation of glycosaminoglycans in the extraocular muscles and in the skin of affected patients. The accumulation of glycosaminoglycans in the skin is a response of local fibroblasts to a stimulating factor in the serum. This substance may block lymphatics and lead to further swelling.[124]

[124]Bull RH, Coburn PR. Pretibial myxoedema: a manifestation of lymphoedema? *Lancet*, 1993, **341**(8842): 403–4.

357

THE FOOT

FOOTWEAR

The shoe may be worn down unevenly, reflecting the gait, or stained by urine or sweat. Alternatively the shoe may mark the foot leading to shoe moulding, callus or ulceration.

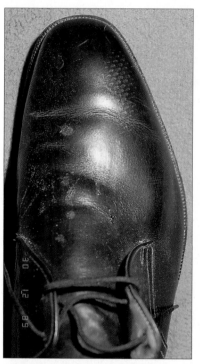

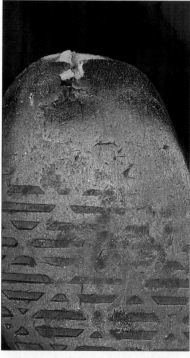

746 The significance of dried urine drops. The shoes may be showered by urine spray. If the urine contains sugar it may dry with a white deposit.

747 Wear of the shoe and gait. Wear that is asymmetrical may reflect the gait. If the sole of the shoe is worn at the toe it may reflect foot drop, while wear on the anterolateral border may reflect circumduction in a hemiparesis. This may allow identification of the owner!

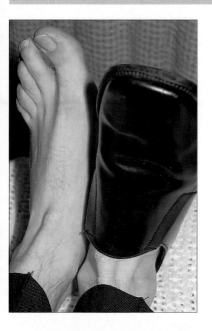

748 Occupational calluses—a chauffeur. This man drove a car with a manual gearbox. If the car had been automatic then one would expect less callus over the left tibialis anterior tendon.

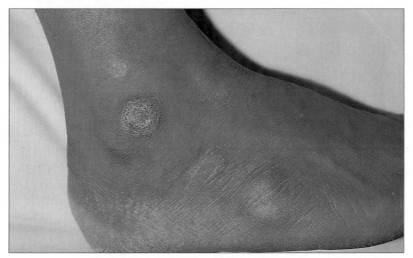

749 Occupational calluses—a Chinese tailor. In many cultures, people sit upon the ground, and sitting on the foot leads to callus over the lateral malleolus and lateral foot. This tailor sat upon the floor to work. A similar callus is seen on those who sit on the foot to pray.

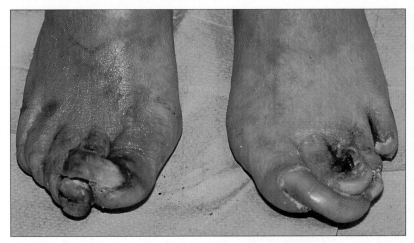

750 The significance of the neglected foot. These nails have not been cut for a year or more, and their length has led to damage. The foot is unwashed. Perhaps this neglect is due to old age, dementia, drug addiction, diabetes mellitus, depression, mental disturbance, blindness, arthritis, or hypothyroidism? Maybe none of these causes are responsible, but the underlying reason will be overlooked unless the clinician asks themself "What is the underlying cause of this neglect?".

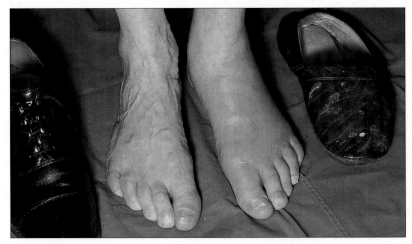

751 Acute gout—the significance of one foot in a slipper. A barrister awoke in the night with unbearable pain in his foot. He came wearing one shoe and a slipper on the painful swollen foot, which would not fit into the shoe—a typical presentation of acute gout.

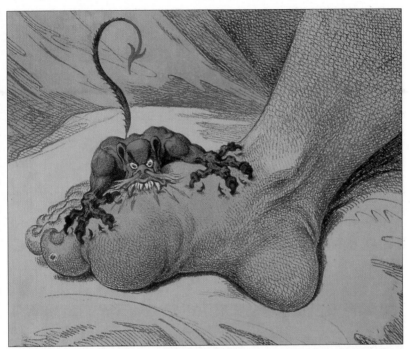

752 Acute gout—the gout devil. This picture of the gouty foot graphically portrays the symptomatology.[125] (Picture originally published by Humphreys in 1794.)

[125]The classic view of gout enshrined in James Gilray's late 18th century cartoon and in subsequent Punch cartoons of the late 19th and early 20th centuries, depicting rich fat old men drinking port in their clubs with a bandaged foot on a gout stool.

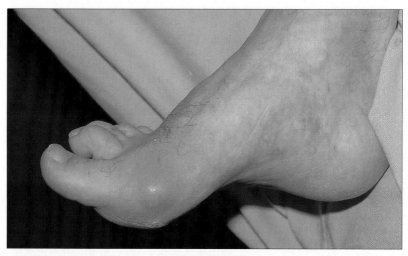

753 Acute gout. This acute monoarthritis on the first postoperative morning after a hernia repair was precipitated by fasting.

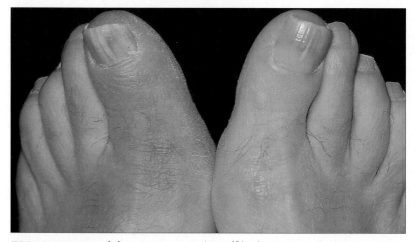

754 Acute gout of the great toe. Podagra,[126] a foot seizure alluding to a man trap, presents overnight as a sudden onset of severe pain in the great toe. It is so exquisitely tender that on waking from sleep even the weight of the sheet cannot be borne. Linear yellow discoloration in the nail of the great toe is due to fungus infection.

---

[126]Etymology: latin and greek, *pous, podos,* foot; *agra,* trap.

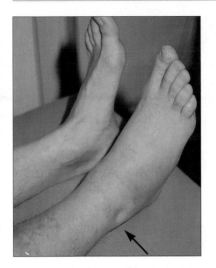

755 Mid-tarsal gout. Gout may affect the mid tarsus and confuse the inexperienced. An American geologist awoke with pain in the mid tarsus, the severity of which convinced him that he must have broken a bone. He referred himself to a radiologist for a radiograph. No firm diagnosis was made for three weeks. Mid-tarsal gout presents as a sudden pain accompanied by oedema, which may be marked and pit on pressure. Crystal (urate) synovitis may be confused with a synovitis due to infection.

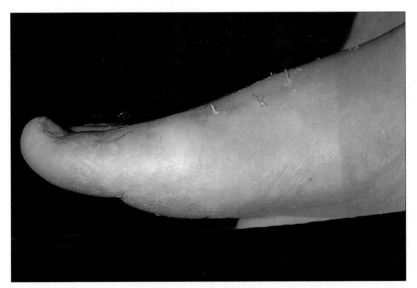

756 An attack of gout subsides. The vivid inflammation and swelling may last 7–14 days and is followed by desquamation. Acute gouty inflammation and acute bacterial inflammation may both desquamate as they remit.

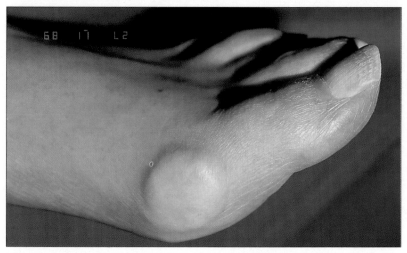

757 A gouty tophus over the first metatarsophalangeal joint. A deposition of urate in a bunion bursa over the first metatarsophalangeal joint.

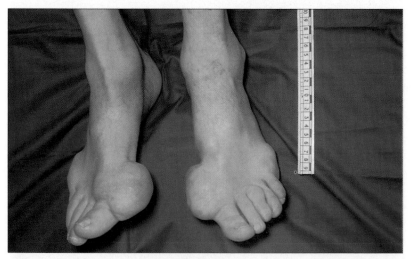

758 Gross tophaceous gout of the feet. Tophi may reach a surprising size around the great toe and be mistaken for osteophytes or bursae. There is a second deposit over the fifth metatarsophalangeal joint. Again a typical colour is seen through the skin (*see* **269**).

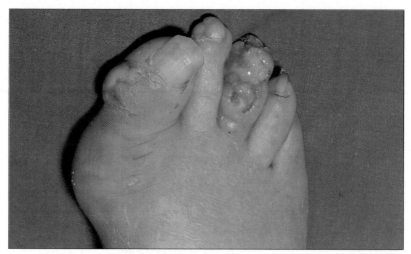

759 Discharging tophi. A tophus overlies the lateral part of the great toe and urate is discharging from a tophus on the middle toe. Treatment for infection was continued for many weeks before the underlying gout was appreciated.

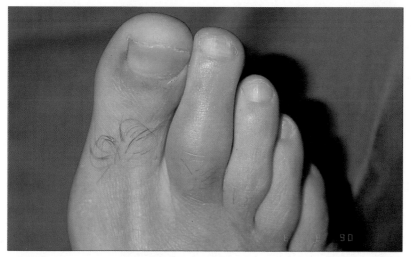

760 The sausage toe. The tenosynovitis of the seronegative arthopathy in **psoriasis** produces the swollen digit (*see* **453**).

RHEUMATOID ARTHRITIS AND CHANGES IN THE FEET

The foot is involved in 80–90% of patients with rheumatoid arthritis. Heel pain may be part of a subcalcaneal or Achilles tendon bursitis or reflect a calcaneal stress fracture. In the forefoot, disease of the metatarsal heads leads to deformity, though initially bursal swelling under weight-bearing areas gives a sensation of walking on pebbles.

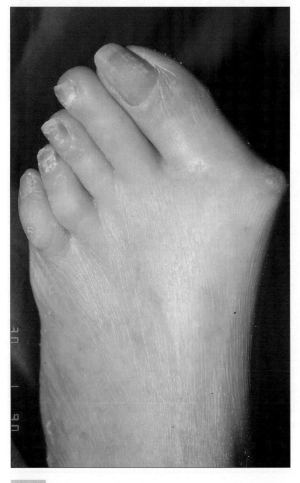

761 Rheumatoid arthritis and fibula drift. Hallux valgus and fibula drift of all the toes

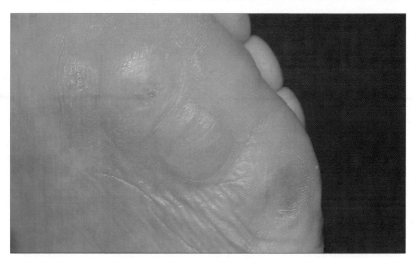

762 Walking on pebbles due to cyst/bursa formation over the metatarsal heads. Discrete swellings over the metatarsal heads are produced by bursitis or cyst formation, leading to a complaint of walking on pebbles. Breakdown of tissue may lead to a fistula and a sinus is seen at the apex of the swelling. Infection may occur.

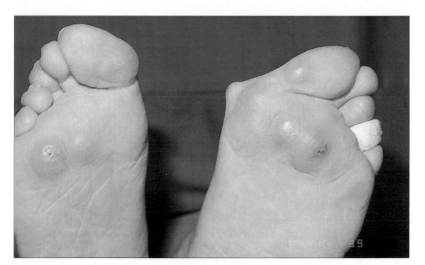

763 Fibula drift nodules and sinus formation. A sinus overlies the bursa associated with the fourth metatarsal heads on both feet. Hallux valgus, metatarsophalangeal subluxation and sinus formation are seen.

DIABETES MELLITUS AND CHANGES IN THE FEET

Diabetic changes in the feet result from:
• infection
• ischaemia
• neuropathy (motor, sensory and autonomic)

Neuropathic joints are a product of the loss of pain sensation and may occur in leprosy, tertiary syphilis (tabes dorsalis) and syringomyelia. In diabetes mellitus there is an additional factor. The autonomic neuropathy and consequent high blood flow due to arterio-venous shunting leads to a warm foot which is osteoporotic with bone which is weak and may collapse in situations of minor stress such as a slip on the pavement kerb. The resultant acute inflammatory episode may lead to rapid joint disorganisation and the production of a neuropathic joint.

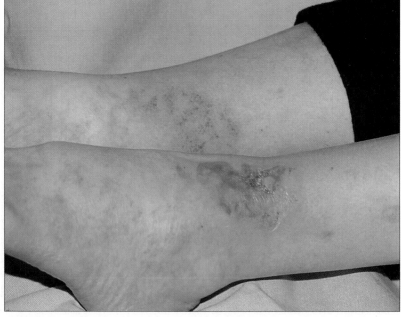

764 The problems of neuropathy and gossip. Painless burns after standing gossiping with the legs by a car exhaust pipe reflect the sensory neuropathy.

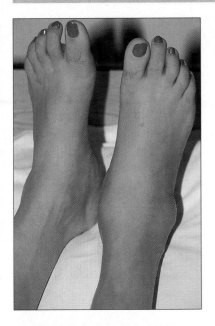

765 Neuropathic ankle joint in diabetes. The changes induced by autonomic neuropathy (the full veins and warm foot result from vascular shunting and reflect the increase flow) are the key to the development of a neuropathic ankle joint in this diabetic with a left hemiplegia. A right subtalar neuropathic ankle joint in the good limb developed after a minor sprain at the kerbside. This led to an osteoporotic trabecular fracture, which started the cycle of joint disorganisation seen here and in **766**.

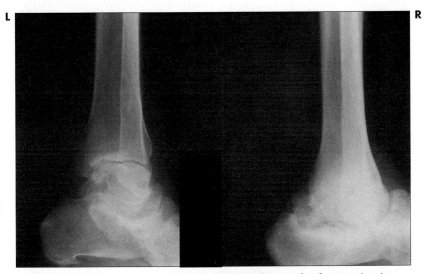

766 Neuropathic ankle joint in a diabetic (radiograph of 765). This shows the joint disorganisation.

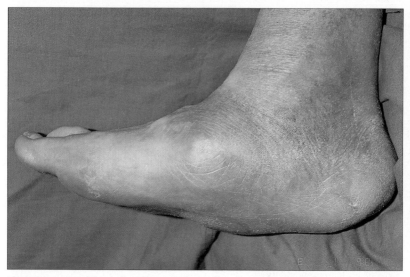

767 Neuropathic rocker-bottom foot. This shows a mid-tarsal rigid rocker-bottom deformity.

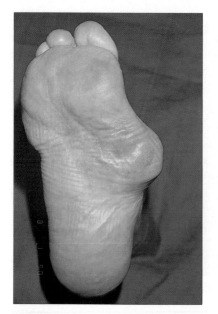

768 Neuropathic mid-tarsal joints. Periodically there is ulceration over the bony points.

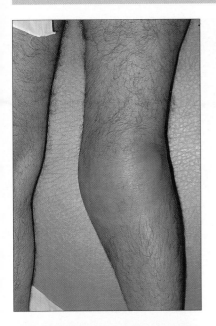

769 Neuropathic knee joint. The knee, in contrast to diabetes mellitus, is the joint most often affected in tabes dorsalis. There is secondary quadriceps wasting. Although painless it has an abnormal range of movement, which leads to further damage.

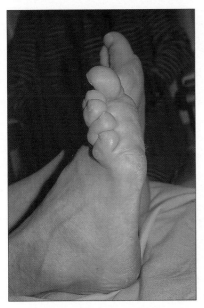

770 Retracted toes. These reflect a tight plantar fascia and weak intrinsic muscles, which lead to clawing of the toes. This can be seen in association with pes cavus.

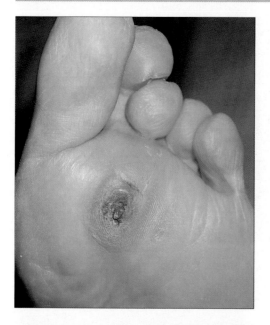

771 Early perforating ulcer of the foot in diabetes mellitus. This 38-year-old woman had a high weight load on the second metatarsal head and bleeding into the callus. Removal showed a perforating ulcer tracking into the interdigital cleft.

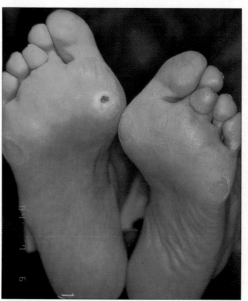

772 Later perforating ulcer in diabetes mellitus. The highly arched diabetic foot with tight plantar fascia has a neuropathic ulcer at a common site over the first metatarsal head. Callus has been removed from over the fifth metatarsal head, which is the other site that is frequently at risk.

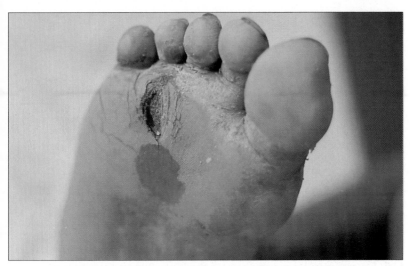

773 Perforating ulcer of the foot in leprosy. Trophic ulcers related to sensory loss are seen in leprosy, but it is over the third metatarsal head, there is no toe retraction and the foot is heavily calloused from walking barefoot.

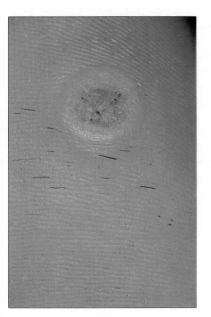

774 The plantar wart. Human papillomaviruses 1 and 2 are the most frequent cause. This wart has a rough keratotic surface surrounded by a smooth collar of thickened keratin. The epidermal ridges are not continued over the surface of the wart. The proliferating tissue is pushed into the subcutaneous tissue and leads to pain. Punctate dark areas are thrombosed capillaries in dermal papillae.

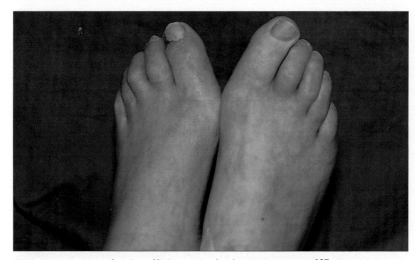

775 Severe vascular insufficiency in the legs—Buerger's[127] sign—1.
Buerger's test demonstrates severe vascular insufficiency. The foot becomes pale when
raised above the level of the heart.

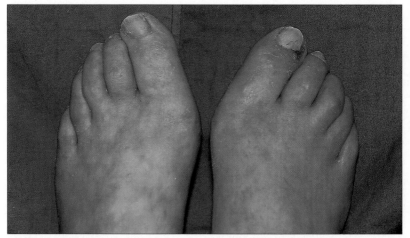

776 Severe vascular insufficiency in the legs—Buerger's sign—2. The foot
becomes mottled when lowered below heart level. There is an ischaemic area at the
base of the great toe.

---

[127]Leo Buerger, US physician, 1879–1943.

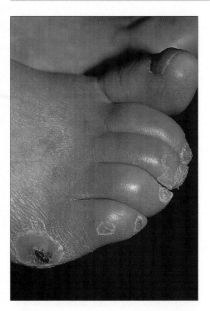

777 Ulceration—sites of danger.
The foot is livid with shiny skin, dystrophic nails and no hair. There is a perforating ulcer at the lateral edge. The three sites of maximum danger are over the lateral and plantar aspect of the foot (fifth metatarsal head and the area under the first metatarsal head, *see* **772**) and around the edge of the heel.

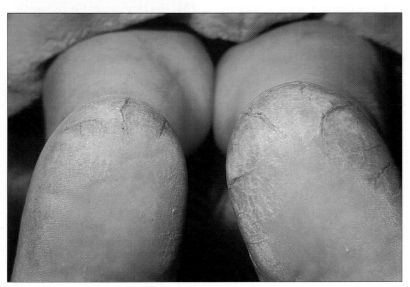

778 Ulceration: sites of danger (2). The cracked callus at the heel border is prone to crack and become ulcerated.

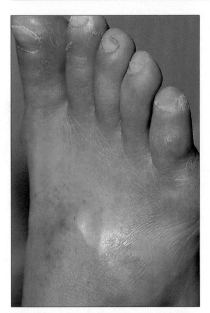

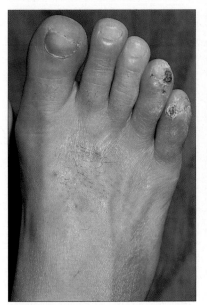

779 The changes of the ischaemic diabetic foot—1. At first it is shiny and mottled.

780 The changes of the ischaemic foot—2. Ischaemic changes then develop at the nail bed.

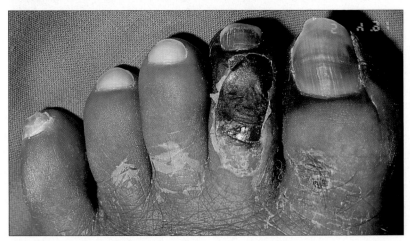

781 The changes of the ischaemic foot—3. The ischaemic changes are followed by gangrene and a demarcation line.

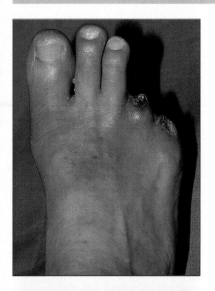

782 The changes of the ischaemic foot—4. Autoamputation may take place along the demarcation line, as happened here in the foot from **779** and **780**.

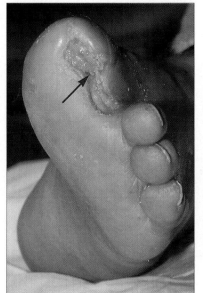

783 The changes of the ischaemic foot—5. Healing may occur. Note the open rigid calcified vessel (arrow).

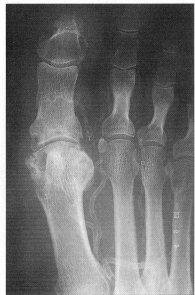

784 Earlier radiograph of forefoot of 783. This shows the pipe-like calcification of the arteries of the same foot.

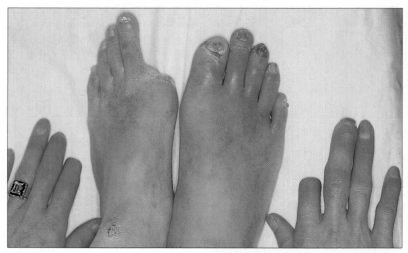

785 Thromboangiitis obliterans—Buerger's disease.[128] This young Chinese male has peripheral vascular disease in both upper and lower limbs. Episodes of thrombophlebitis may recur. The relationship with smoking forms part of the syndrome. In this case he continued to smoke and grasped the cigarette between the proximal phalanges because the distal ones were lost!

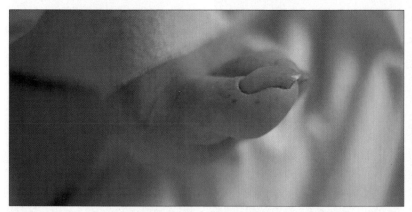

786 Emboli in skin of the toes. Emboli of this size are indistinguishable from purpura. In this case of bacterial endocarditis a proximal aneurysm should be suspected (*see* **716b**).

---

[128]Buerger L. Thromboangiitis obliterans; a study of the vascular lesions leading to presenile spontaneous gangrene. *Am. J. Med.*, 1908, **136**: 567–80.

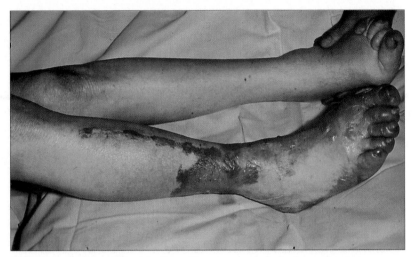

787 An acute arterial embolism. There is an embolus in the popliteal artery. Initially the leg became painful, pale, paraesthetic, paralysed, pulseless and then perishing cold (**PPPPPP**—the six P's).It progresses from white to dusky blue after 4–5 hours and finally, as seen here, to a fixed blue/black mottling. Then it is irreversibly ischaemic.The cause may be thrombotic, embolic or related to an underlying disease such as diabetes or a connective tissue disorder.

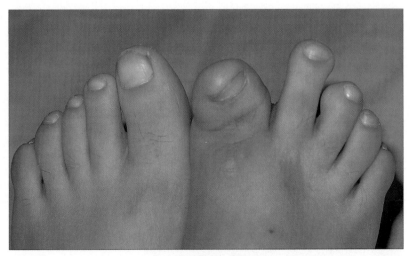

788 The short toe. This is a clue to **sickle cell disease**. After the initial bone crisis with infarction, which usually occurs in childhood, the phalanx may shorten.

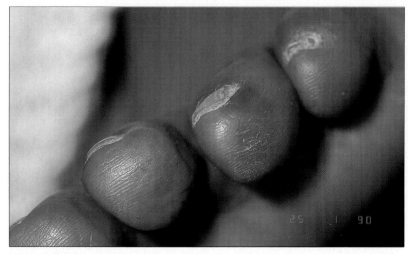

789 Chilblains (perniosis). A tourist from the Arabian gulf came to London in mid January during a university term break. Shopping in sandals in Bond street led to pain and itch in the tips of the toes so she bought fur-lined boots! Chilblains are a cold-induced ischaemia, which is secondary to a combination of tight clothing impeding the circulation and poor insulation. There is a cutaneous vasculitis with the liberation of histamine, inflammation and ischaemia. Tight jeans or jodhpurs and the insulation of fat legs may lead to chilblains on the thighs.

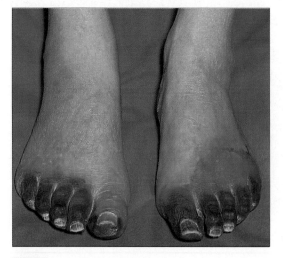

790 Frost bite. More severe cold injury is a risk for every polar explorer if inadequately protected. This shows gangrene of all the toes secondary to cold injury in an alcoholic male who spent a November night on a bench on the London embankment using newspapers to cover his trunk to keep warm. He has frost bite aggravated by an impaired arterial circulation. A line of demarcation with erythema is present.

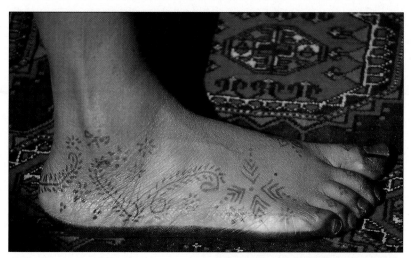

791 The hennaed foot. Henna (*see* **364**) has been used here as decoration and to toughen the skin. Patterns of great intricacy may be seen.

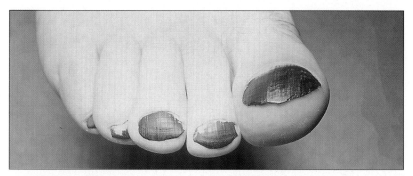

792 'Nigranychia'. Always get the patient's confidence and he will tell you the answers. The black nail is the result of soaking the feet in a patent medicine containing potassium permanganate. This man (a publican who drank excessive alcohol) developed a burning sensation in his feet. His doctor arranged an outpatient appointment at a liver unit, but meanwhile the feet became unbearable. He sat drinking in the evening, with his feet in the patent medicine and the potassium permanganate reacted with the keratin, dying the skin dark brown. Before his appointment he scrubbed off the skin, but could not dislodge the potassium permanganate from the nails—hence 'nigranychia'. A silly story, but the patient went to the MRCP examination, and though the abdomen showed hepatosplenomegaly and a liver biopsy puncture, the nails caused a lot of anxious moments for the candidates.

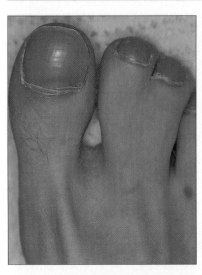

793 Clubbed cyanosed toenails.
The toenails may show less marked
change than the fingernails, perhaps due
to the effect of shoe moulding (see page
238 for a full discussion). The second and
third toe are webbed.

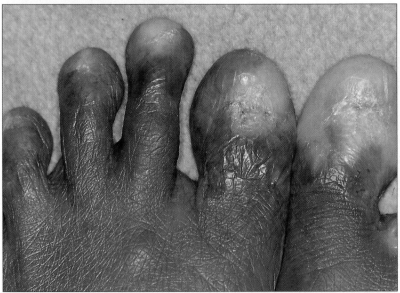

794 Destruction of the nail bed—lichen planus. Nail destruction may be due to
barefoot football or intrinsic disease. In lichen planus changes range from longitudinal
ridging to loss of the nail. The cuticle has grown over it leading to pterygium unguis and
permanent nail loss.

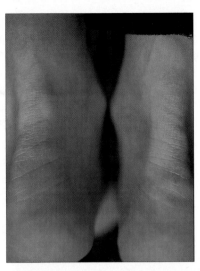

795a Tendon xanthomas. A dentist complained of pain in the Achilles tendon. The fusiform swellings are tendon xanthomas, which are local infiltrates of lipid-rich histiocyte foam cells. They are the hallmark of familial hypercholesterolaemia.

795b. Eruptive xanthomas. Eruptive xanthomas on the skin may be seen in familial hypercholesterolaemia. In women with secondary hypercholesterolaemia it is particularly important to exclude hypothyroidism.

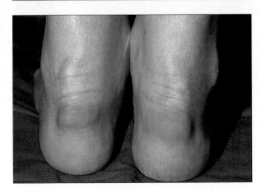

796 Heel xanthomas. The hard heel swelling may be mistaken for tophi or rheumatic nodules. It may become inflamed and mimic Achilles tenosynovitis, particularly in the athlete.

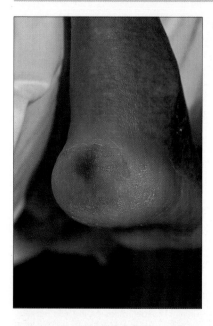

797 The heel as a pressure point. This pressure sore on the prominence of the calcaneum caused by pressure while lying immobile on a trolley will break down.

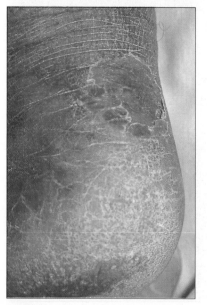

798 Shoe rub at the heel. The pressure sore shown in **797** is at a different level from the rub produced by the edge of a shoe, which may precipitate ulceration in the diabetic.

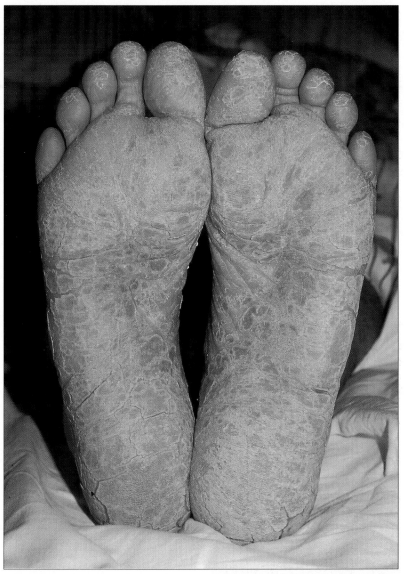

799 Hyperkeratosis of the soles due to practolol (*see* 387). Hyperkeratosis of the soles may be due to friction and the effect of walking barefoot, tylosis, a congenital defect, a drug reaction or psoriasis.

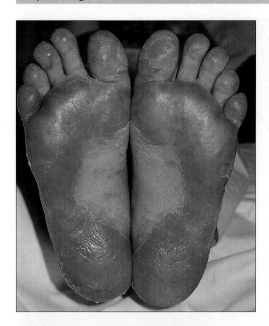

800 Stevens–Johnson syndrome and the sole. Exfoliation of the soles of the feet is seen in the Stevens–Johnson syndrome. The associated tenderness may preclude walking (*see* **297**).

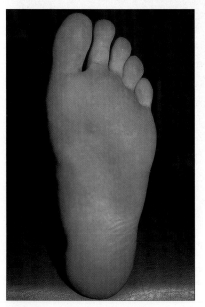

801 Plantar erythema. This may coexist with palmar erythema and have the same associations (*see* **388**). Do not confuse with erythromelalgia, which is characterised by painful red hot extremities associated with thrombocythaemia and relieved by aspirin. Primary erythromelalgia is first seen in childhood, is bilateral and symmetrical, and is aggravated by exercise and warmth. Secondary erythromelalgia occurs in gout and in collagen disease (systemic lupus erythematosus and polyarteritis nodosa) and is not associated with any platelet dysfunction.

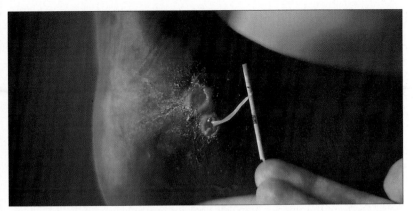

802 The guinea worm (*Dracunculus medinensis*). The 'fiery serpent' emerges. Infection results from drinking from unprotected ground water sources containing the minute crustacean vector infected with the third-stage larvae, which are released in the stomach to mature, migrate and mate. The gravid female then emerges, usually on an extremity, secreting a substance from her vulva that induces a blister from which the eggs emerge: this is often synchronous with the rainy season. Worms become lost and calcify; they may be palpated under the skin and seen on radiographs. The main complication is sepsis.

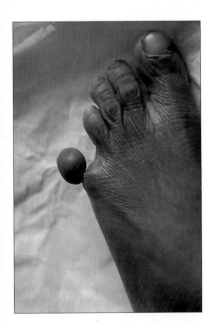

803 Ainhum. This Nigerian farmer's only complaint was of pain in the foot if it was knocked. A constricting band around the base of the little toe may deepen and lead to autoamputation. This is common in Africa, and the differential diagnosis includes leprosy and other neuropathies, systemic sclerosis and rare palmar–plantar keratoderma. Pseudo-ainhum may occur secondary to another condition.

THE EXTENSOR PLANTAR RESPONSE (BABINSKI RESPONSE[129]).

The extensor plantar response is the classic sign of an upper motor neurone lesion. Suspect it if the patient trips over paving stones or the carpet and when testing tone, by rolling the leg (external/internal rotation at the hip), if it is increased. Elicit it with a blunt, pointed object such as a key by stroking the lateral edge of the foot firmly. Warn the patient about what you are going to do and watch closely. In an early lesion the upgoing toe may only appear once or twice and then you will be in the doubtful area of "The plantars are equivocal!", a common situation in clinical practice. It is analogous to the statement "I am absolutely certain that I can feel the spleen/hear a murmur etc.," when what is meant is the exact opposite "I am not sure if…"

Next look for a level. Remember that the lesion can be anywhere from the motor cortex to the anterior horn cell. Look for reflex changes. If the leg tendon reflexes are absent the cord lesion must be combined with a neuropathy.

Absent ankle jerks with upgoing toes occur in:

- Taboparesis.
- Friedreich's ataxia.
- Subacute combined degeneration of the cord.
- A conus or lower cord lesion.

Conversely, absent ankle jerks and downgoing toes occur in:

- A neuropathy.
- An L5–S1 root lesion.

---

[129]Joseph Francois Felix Babinski, French neurologist, 1857–1932.

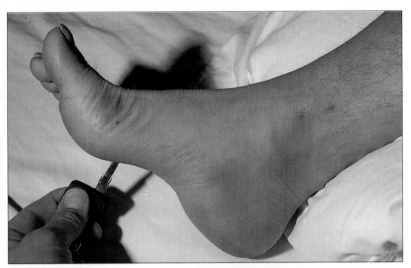

804 The extensor plantar response (a Babinski response). There is gross extension of the great toe at the metacarpophalangeal joint while the other toes may fan.

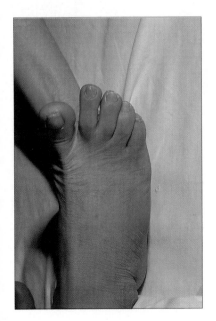

805 The extensor plantar response (the dorsal view). The other toes may fan and dorsiflex. This response may also be elicited by firm pressure on the shin and a downstroke to the foot. It indicates a disturbance of the function, but not necessarily structure, of the pyramidal tracts, and is seen in most cases of coma.

KAPOSI'S SARCOMA

This is seen:
- In elderly males as a sporadic condition unassociated with human immuno-deficiency virus (HIV).
- In Sub-Saharan Africa as an endemic condition before the advent of HIV.
- In association with HIV and acquired immune deficiency syndrome (AIDS) as an epidemic condition, specially among homosexuals (*see* **328**).
- As an iatrogenic condition in association with immunosuppression in organ transplantation.

All types of Kaposi's sarcoma have in common the presence of herpes virus like DNA fragments in the abnormal tissue.[130]

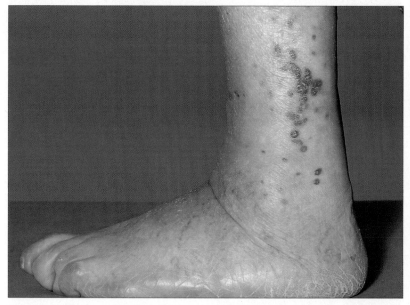

806 The elderly male of Mediterranean descent. An incidental problem during an admission for bronchopneumonia. The purple plaques on the legs are indolent. There is a little oedema. This is sporadic Kaposi's sarcoma.

---

[130]Moore PS, Chang Y. Detection of herpesvirus–like DNA sequences in Kaposi's sarcoma in patients with and without HIV infection. *New England Journal of Medicine*, 1995, **332**(18): 1181–5.

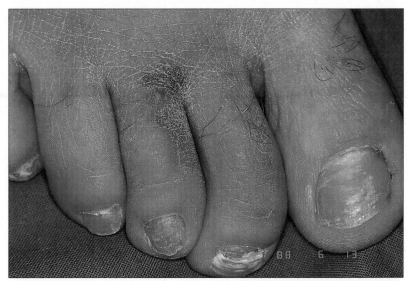

807 The HIV-positive male.[131] This man is a professional *athlete*. He has young feet, but they are dry, with a pustule in a follicle on both third and fourth toes. He also has onycholysis of all nails, and a purple plaque between the second and third toes, which is epidemic Kaposi's sarcoma.

---

[131]This man is a ballet dancer. Young feet should be moist. If they are dry there is an underlying neuropathy or there has been a re-emergence of eczema, which is so often seen in acquired immune deficiency syndrome (AIDS). It is unusual to have a pustule on healthy young feet and this is a sign of immunosuppression, diabetes mellitus or AIDS as a result of depressed neutrophil function with an opsonisation defect. Onycholysis is due to the trauma of dance or a fungal infection, which can result from a loss of T cell-mediated immunity and therefore an increased susceptibility to dermatophytic infection. *Opportunist infections hunt in packs!*

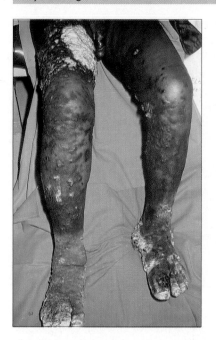

808 The HIV-negative African.
There are widespread flat-topped plaques, coalescing in places and further disguised by calamine lotion. This is endemic Kaposi's sarcoma.

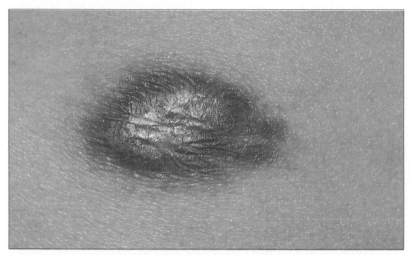

809 The classic plaque of Kaposi's sarcoma in the white skin. The dark red plaque appears blacker on black skin, as do so many red rashes.

THE SKIN

PRURITUS

Itching provokes scratching, which leaves marks on the accessible skin. Skin rashes may itch. Pruritus without skin lesions may be due to local or generalised causes, many of which are metabolic.

- Generalised skin diseases that cause pruritus include parasitic infestation, eczema, miscellaneous conditions such as lichen planus, urticaria, dermatitis, and dermatitis herpetiformis, and senile eczema.
- Internal diseases causing generalised itching include cholestasis , diabetes mellitus, thyroid disease, renal failure, blood disease, bronchial carcinoma and lymphoma.
- Local itch occurs in diabetes mellitus around the vulva, in contact sensitivity and in pruritus ani.

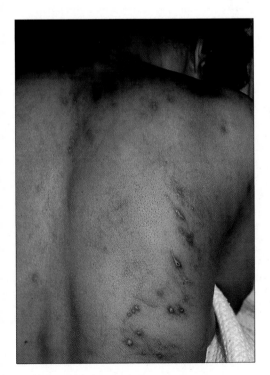

810 Marks on the back only where it is accessible. The excoriations are all on parts which can be reached and may be seen in cholestasis (even before jaundice), in renal failure and in diabetes mellitus. Buffed nails give a clue (*see* **472**). Itch may be due to a drug reaction and is a feature of cocaine addiction.

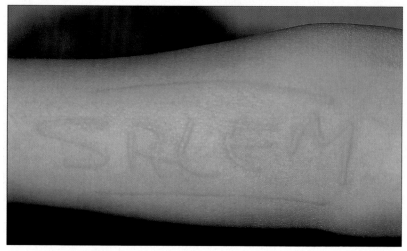

811 Dermographism. In some individuals scratching produces excessive wheals due to the liberation of histamine and may be part of a chronic urticaria. This boy had attacks of recurrent facial swelling. The initial blanching flare and developing wheal reflect the dermographic appearance of this dramatic triple response.

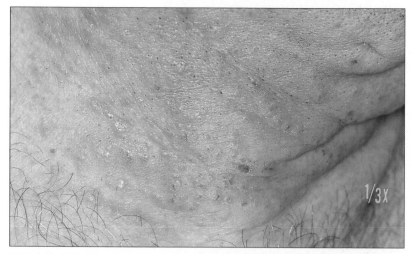

812 Itch in leukaemia. Itch may be due to blood dyscrasias such as leukaemia, polycythaemia rubra vera, and iron deficiency anaemia. The mechanical trauma leads to thickening of the skin.

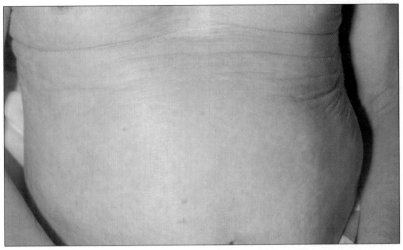

813 Itch in Hodgkin's disease. The 'itchy' skin may be actually infiltrated by deposits of lymphoma.

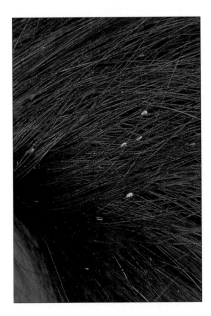

814 Egg cases in the hair. The 'itchy' skin may contain parasites. Scabies may be difficult to confirm in the early stages and the burrows difficult to find (*see* **385**). Nits in the scalp are less easy to see than the egg cases attached at scalp level to the hair, which then move away from the scalp with hair growth.

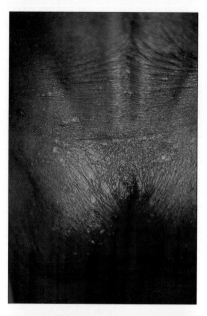

815 Nodularity in onchocerciasis.
In the skin the parasites of onchocerciasis provoke intense pruritus. The red fresh blood on the left sacrum is the site of a diagnostic skin snip.

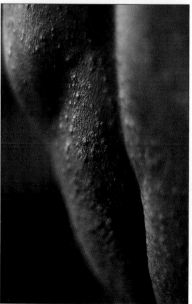

816 Lichenification in onchocerciasis. The intense pruritus leads to lichenification and a leather-like skin, which hangs in folds.

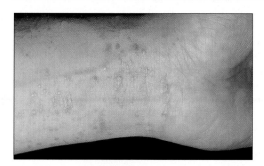

817 Itchy wrists due to lichen planus. Lichen planus may produce itching at the wrist and ankles and its presence suggests that other areas should be examined (*see* **315**, **677**, **743**).

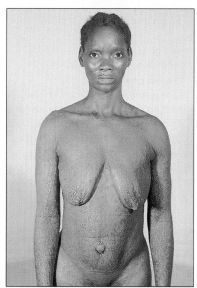

818 Lichen planus on the trunk. The lichenification may be extensive.

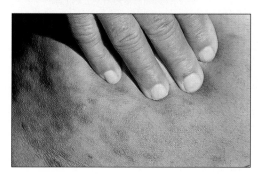

819 Lichen planus and even buffed nails. Lichen planus also leads to lichenification of the mauve flat-topped shiny papules.

THOUGHT PROCESSES IN RASHES

Listen and look–then ask yourself "Why is it like that?". How does its distribution reflect life, light or contact with the environment? Remember that skin diseases, though legion, usually fall into one of these areas: acne; bacteriological ,viral and fungal infections; tumours; dermatitis; psoriasis; leg ulcers and warts.

Age and race will make some conditions more likely. Distribution may vary over the body:

- Hands and feet in contact dermatitis
- Face and flexures in atopy
- Face, chest and groin in seborrhoeic dermatitis
- On the legs in gravity associated immune complex deposition
- On the periphery in erythema multiforme
- On exposed areas in ultra-violet light sensitivity
- On the wrists and fingerwebs, and around the nipples in scabies
- On the pressure areas—knee, elbow, sacrum—in psoriasis.

Symmetry is usual in the endogenous conditions, whereas fleas bite randomly. If the rash is of incongruous distribution, then think again. Look all over for a typical lesion, as much of the rash may have been modified by scratching or infection. Shape may be helpful, with rings indicating annular lesions of lichen planus or fungus, linear forms in a dermatome distribution showing herpes zoster and facial haemangiomata, or no dermatome distribution in isomorphic trauma (the Koebner phenomenon of linear rashes in relation to sites of trauma). The examples on these two pages show how thought can lead to diagnosis.

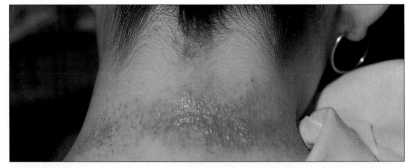

820 The teenager and a sore neck. Nickel is a very common sensitiser, and is usually present as a plating or an alloy in jewellery and fasteners of clothing. It is ubiquitous—small amounts are even found in detergents. Since contact dermatitis can mimic most eruptions, diagnosis requires suspicion and a careful history. The distribution is valuable. This eczematous rash affects the necklace area, ear lobes and wrist (*see* **386**).

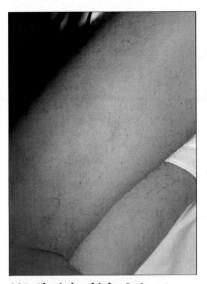

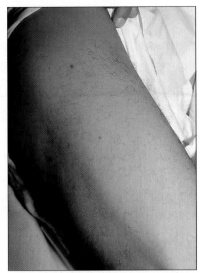

821 The itchy thigh—1. Sometimes the sensitiser may be less clear, but analysis leads to diagnosis. A patch of itchy eczema on the left thigh—but if this is simple eczema it should be bilateral and symmetrical and yet the right thigh is clear (*see* **822**).

822 The itchy thigh—2. The rash shown in **821** is not bilateral as the right thigh is clear. A contact sensitivity is therefore possible and the area lies under the trouser pocket.

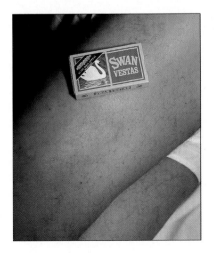

823 The itchy thigh—3. This right-handed smoker keeps his red-tipped 'strike anywhere' matches in his left trouser pocket. The **phosphorus sesquisulphide** in the matches has leached through and the phosphorus has sensitised the skin.

EIGHTEENTH CENTURY ARTEFACTS AND MODERN MEDICINE

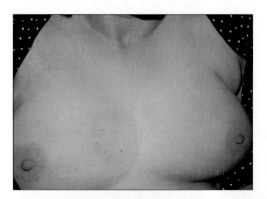

824 Chest pain—differential diagnosis. This is a reaction to the adhesive of electrocardiogram electrodes and is a marker of cardiac monitoring in intensive care. It could be assumed that recent monitoring has been performed, but a similar appearance can be produced by care in the community (*see* **825**).

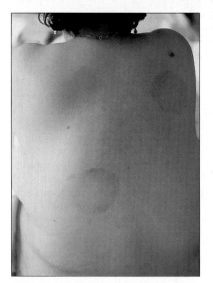

825 Dry cupping. This appearance is produced by applying a glass cup, which has been momentarily flamed with a taper, to the skin, where it has been stuck by suction. This is a treatment for fever and is sometimes modified by previous scarification of the skin to allow dark venous blood to be sucked out (*see* **826**).

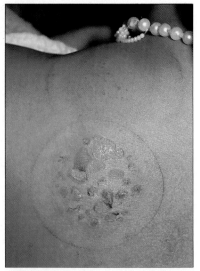

826 Wet cupping. This is cupping (*see* **825**) with previous scarification of the skin to allow dark venous blood to be sucked out and so allow the 'noxious toxins' escape—a potent folk remedy.

CHILDHOOD RASHES

Childhood rashes may appear in the adult. Their appearance is mimicked by drug rashes and used as a descriptive term (e.g. morbilliform, 'like measles').

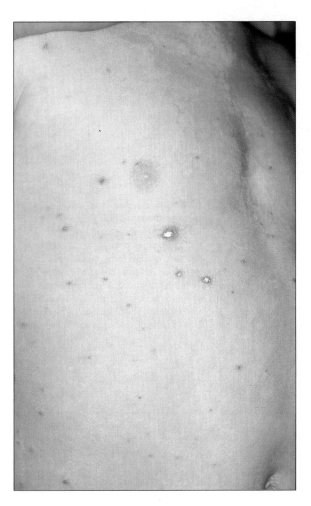

827 Chickenpox in childhood. The rash is concentrated on the trunk. It consists of macules, papules and vesicles, and all these morphologies are present at the same time. Calamine lotion causes the white marks.

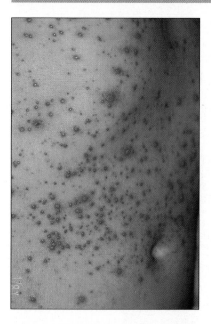

828 Chickenpox in the immunosuppressed adult. In the adult, chickenpox may be more severe than in childhood and the systemic upset can be considerable.

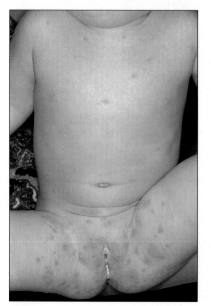

829 Chickenpox and its distribution. The distribution of the varicella virus is centripetal in contrast to that of smallpox and erythema multiforme. It is seen on covered areas of the body more than the exposed cooler ones, here being denser in the area of the nappy and sparser over the abdomen and trunk, which had not been covered. The eruption is present in all its stages.

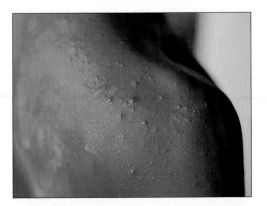

830 Chickenpox on a black skin. On a pigmented skin the rash may be overlooked, the vesicles appearing as a few drops of water on the surface.

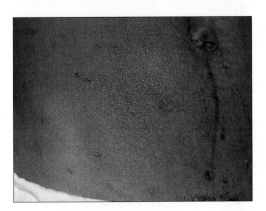

831 Chickenpox on a brown skin. The rash may be sparse in an adult, but remains polymorphic and has a centripetal distribution.

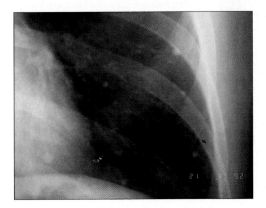

832 Chickenpox residua on the chest radiograph. Chickenpox may affect the lung resulting in secondary infection and a severe bronchopneumonia. Other features can include hepatitis, encephalitis and purpura fulminans. The residual benign nodular calcifications are seen on radiography.

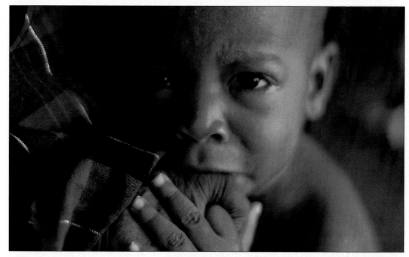

833 Measles and misery. The child infected with this paramyxovirus (a single strand of ribonucleic acid) after an incubation of 10 days is miserable and seeks solace. There is a mild conjunctivitis and an early maculopapular rash on the forehead.

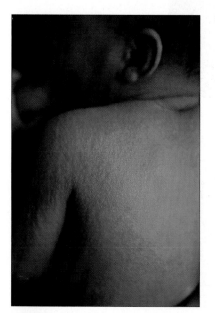

834 Measles rash on a black skin. The rash, generated by a cell mediated response, becomes widespread, especially over the back. Papules coalesce to produce a thick furry appearance to the skin, which has a dark red colour. In the lower part, normal skin is seen between the rash. On a white skin the rash is red; upon a black skin it is much darker.

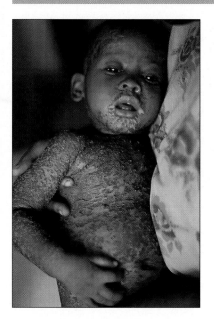

835 Peeling measles rash. After a further 10 days the rash peels and a browny desquamation takes place. If this is severe large plaques of skin flake off. By this stage the exanthem has led to profound immunosuppression and may precipitate diarrhoea, pneumonia and the illness of kwashiorkor. This child has angular stomatitis. The chance of death in the year after measles is increased by a factor of 10.

836 Rubella. Many rashes produced by viral infections are similar in appearance. It is easy to mistake German measles—rubella caused by an enveloped RNA virus—for another virus infection such as infectious mononucleosis. If it is also complicated by an arthritis it may be confused with mumps or viral hepatitis. The rash is maculopapular with sparse spots 1–4 mm in size.

837 Rubella. The rash appears first on the cheeks, spreads to the trunk and limbs, and coalesces. Lymph node enlargement, particularly of the suboccipital and cervical lymph nodes, is a constant finding, but the mucous membrane of the mouth is clean compared to the redness and Koplik spots of measles. A few flecks of exudate may be seen on the tonsils. The conjunctivae may be a faint pink. It is essential to investigate the woman presenting with suspected infection in early pregnancy.

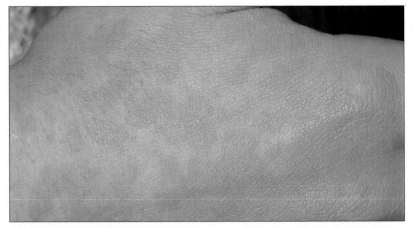

838 Infectious mononucleosis. The rash induced by ampicillin inadvertently used in infectious mononucleosis in comparison to that of rubella, which it resembles, although rubella is less florid (see **334**).

ERYTHEMA MULTIFORME AND RINGS

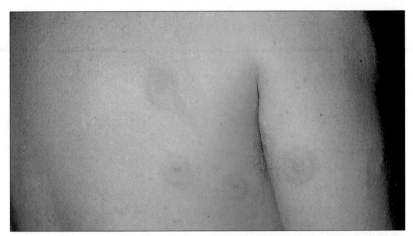

839 Erythema multiforme (*see* 297, 381). This often begins as a red plaque. It has a predilection for the periphery and is a reaction to a panoply of stimuli. In this man genital herpes one week earlier was followed by the appearance of these red plaques up to 1 cm in diameter.

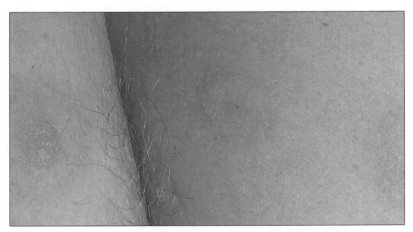

840 Erythema iris. In erythema multiforme, the variant rashes bear descriptive names. The target lesion is erythema iris, a central vesicle with a clear area and an erythematous ring around it. The lesions may be vesicles, bullae, macules or papules—in fact multiform.

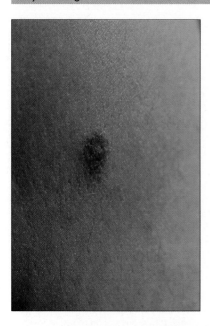

841 Erythema iris. In this ageing lesion there has been some bleeding into the vesicle and it has darkened.

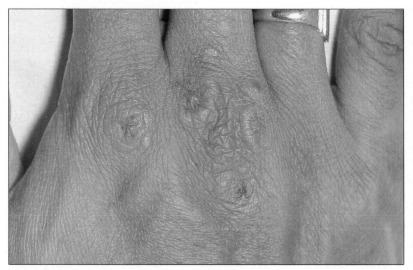

842 Erythema iris. Lesions frequently appear on the limbs and classically on the back of the hands.

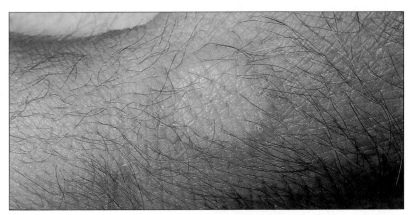

843 Tinea as a target lesion. Tinea corporis produces the characteristic appearance of annular ringworm. The active scaly edge contrasts with the inactive central zone and may reflect immunological changes as antigens diffusing from hyphae in the stratum corneum are presented to the immune system by the epidermal Langerhans' cells. Cellular immunity is of paramount importance in the defence against dermatophytes and accounts for the high incidence of these infections in the acquired immune deficiency syndrome (AIDS).

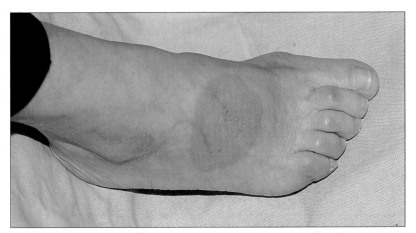

844 Granuloma annulare. Focal inflammation of collagen with inflammation and fibrosis characterises the necrobiotic disorders, which include necrobiosis lipoidica and granuloma annulare. Both have an association with diabetes mellitus. Granuloma annulare affects young adults and consists of a ring of closely grouped papules, commonly on the dorsum of the feet or hands.

409

THE SKIN AND THE GUT

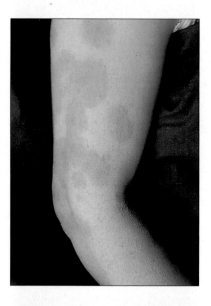

845 Pyoderma gangrenosum—the spectrum—1 (*see* 704). This is characterised by a necrotising, destructive, non-infective skin ulceration. It may begin as an erythematous area with some nodularity, as in this woman with ulcerative colitis.

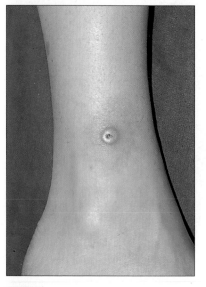

846 Pyoderma gangrenosum—the spectrum—2. The erythematous area may develop a sterile pustule.

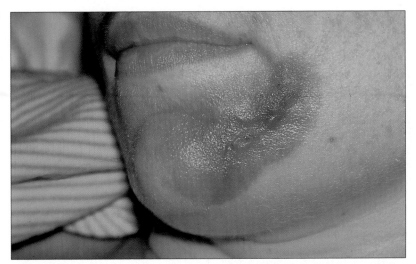

847 Pyoderma gangrenosum–the spectrum—3. The lesion then becomes red or violet.

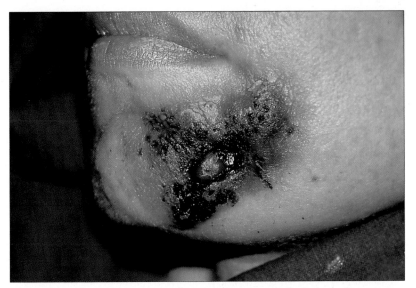

848 Pyoderma gangrenosum–the spectrum—4. Finally the lesion becomes necrotic. The face and leg are common sites (*see* **704**). It heals leaving a papery scar (*see* **705**).

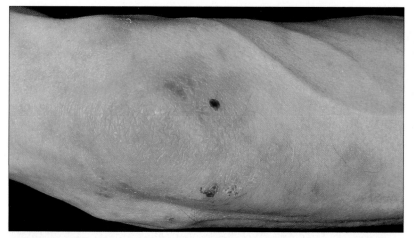

849 Dermatitis herpetiformis on the back of the elbow. An intensely itchy recurrent dermatitis which may be concentrated at typical sites: the extensor surface of the knees and elbows, the dorsum of the shoulder and the pelvic girdle. The scalp and hands may show scattered lesions.

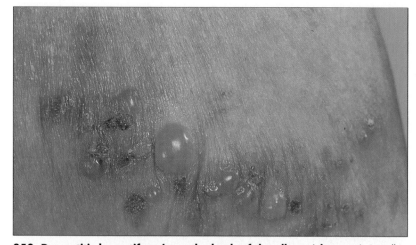

850 Dermatitis herpetiformis on the back of the elbow (close-up). Initially starting as red papules and wheals, clustered small blisters of varied shape and size and of symmetrical distribution appear. Histology shows eosinophils and granular deposits of IgA and C_3 in dermal papillae. Associated with gluten enteropathy, it responds to treatment with diaminodiphenyl sulphone (dapsone), sulphapyriadine and a gluten free diet. Many patients are first thought to have scabies.

PSORIASIS

Psoriasis is a common genetically determined chronic skin disease characterised by sharply demarcated red plaques, which are particularly seen on the knees, elbows, scalp, sacrum and penis. There is enormous morphological variation. Nail changes may occur. It may be complicated by joint disease.

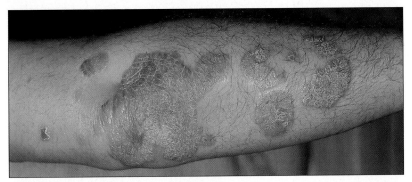

851 Psoriasis—discoid or nummular. The red plaques have silvery scales and frequently develop at sites of trauma or scars. The isomorphic response is also known as the Koebner[132] phenomenon, a development of skin disease at sites of trauma which is also seen in lichen planus, active eczema, and molluscum contagiosum

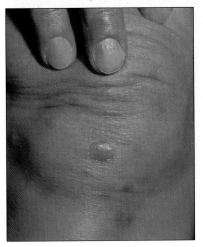

852 Guttate psoriasis. Small 0.5–1.0 cm lesions seen as red, slightly scaly, spots like drops over the skin, while the nail shows pitting. It may follow a streptococcal sore throat.

---

[132]Heinrich Koebner, German dermatologist, 1838–1904.

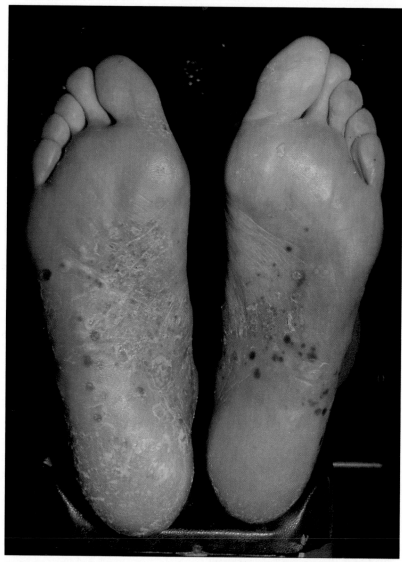

853 Pustular psoriasis. A name used when pustules are present. Red and scaly plaques develop—often symmetrically—on the palms and soles in association with rupioid/limpet-like lesions. It is often limited to the hands, the thenar and hypothenar eminences and on the instep and lateral border (**854**) of the feet.

LEPROSY

Leprosy, a chronic infectious disease caused by Mycobacterium Leprae, which affects the peripheral nerves and skin. It is a great mimic whose spectrum of appearance reflects the two extremes of host reaction, from an almost complete lack of resistance to one of effective host immunity. It can, for example, imitate:-

- Vitiligo
- Fungus infections
- Cutaneous tuberculosis,
- Systemic lupus erythematosus,
- Leishmaniasis
- Kaposi's sarcoma
- Birthmarks
- Common skin conditions such as oncocerciasis

Though rarely seen in Europe, it is common world wide and there should be a high degree of suspicion if it is not to be overlooked.

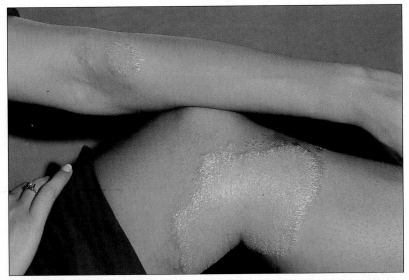

854 Tuberculoid leprosy versus lupus pernio. Tuberculoid leprosy is stable, presenting with a skin lesion associated with nerve involvement, often with thickening of unnamed cutaneous nerves. The original presentation of this patient in a sarcoidosis clinic was due to the chronic granulomatous histology. However, these hypopigmented plaques with a red raised border were insensitive to pin prick and there was thickening of some peripheral nerves. Contrast this with **855**.

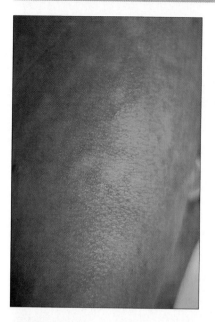

855 Lepromatous leprosy. This is characterised by erythematous skin lesions with macule formation in the skin in association with raised patchy areas of depigmentation.

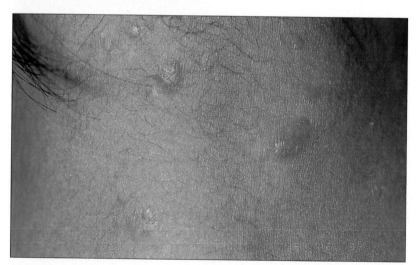

856 Lupus pernio. These raised purple plaques on the back of the neck are the clue to the nature of the chronic lung disease, which was treated for nine months as tuberculosis. They showed sarcoid granulomas on biopsy.

BLEEDING INTO THE SKIN

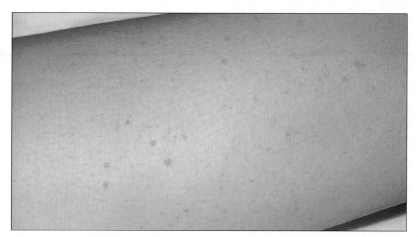

857 Purpura. Bleeding into the skin leads to purple spots, which do not blanch on pressure and vary in size from pinhead-size, as here, to larger areas (*see* **858**).

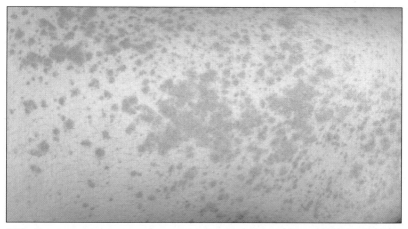

858 Purpura. Larger areas of purpura in contrast to those shown in **857**. Purpura may be due to a deficiency of platelets (thrombocytopenic purpura), a vascular defect, vasculitis or a disorder of coagulation. Remember scurvy with capillary fragility and the purpura of old age. Purpura is more common in the legs due to the relative increase in hydrostatic pressure.

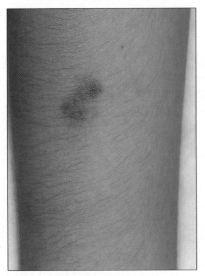

859 A bruise. As the blood is broken down it follows a characteristic colour cycle.

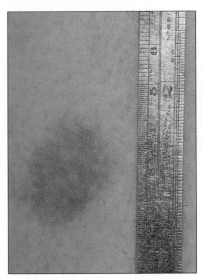

860 A fading bruise.. This shows colour changes from red to purple to yellow to brown and then fades.

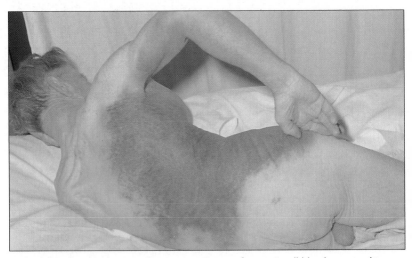

861 A big bruise in a patient on anticoagulants. Small bleeds or petechiae may coalesce to form ecchymoses.

ENDPIECE

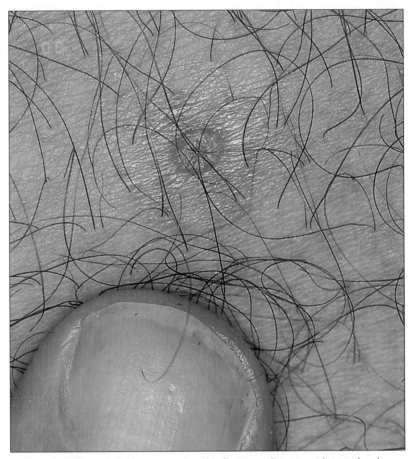

862 The eschar scar of Tsutsugamushi disease. This man took a weekend break on a small deserted island in the Dutch East Indies. He had several insect bites. On his return he developed a severe fever, headache, prostration and renal failure. Despite commenting on the black spot on his thigh no one looked at it. He received large doses of ototoxic antibiotics and developed severe vestibular symptoms. Many cases of **scrub typhus** may go undiagnosed if the eschar is overlooked and the treatment offered may be worse than the disease. Rickettsia tsutsugamushi infects larval mites when they feed on rodents, and the human gets bitten when he interposes himself between the two.

Movement	Muscle	Weakness in UMN lesion	Root	UMN reflex change	Nerve
shoulder abduct	deltoid	++	C5		axillary
elbow flexion	biceps		C5/6	biceps	musculocutaneous
	brachioradialis		C6	supinator	radial
elbow extension	triceps	+	C7	triceps	radial
radial wrist extension	ext. carp. rad.	+	C6		radial
finger extension	ext. dig.	+	C7	(+)	post interosseus
finger flexion	flex. poll. long. and flex. dig. prof. index f. d. p. ring + little		C8	+	ant interosseus
finger abduction	1st dorsal inteross.	++	T1		ulnar
	abductor poll. brev.	++	T1		median
hip flexion	iliopsoas	++	L1/2	+	femoral
hip adduction	adductors		L2/3		obturator
hip extension	gluteus maximus		L5/S1		sciatic
knee flexion	hamstrings		S1	++	sciatic
knee extension	quadriceps		L3/4		femoral
ankle dorsiflexion	tibialis anterior	++	L4		deep peroneal
ankle eversion	peroneii		L5/S1	++	superior peroneal
ankle plantarflex	gastroc./soleus		S1/S2		tibial
big toe extension	extensor hall. long.		L5		deep peroneal

Colours reflect common cord segments

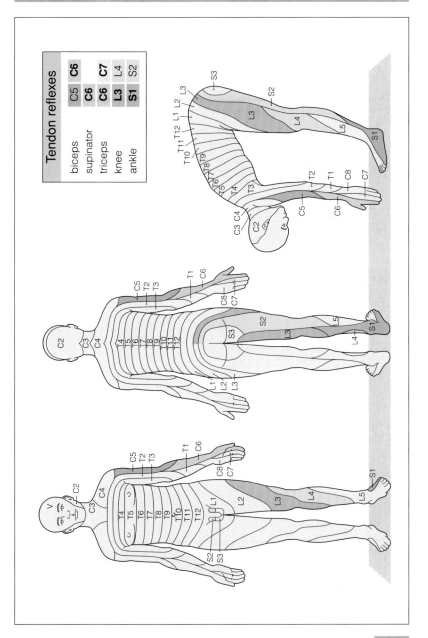

Index

References printed in medium type are to page numbers (e.g. 123), those in bold are to picture and caption numbers (e.g. **123**), while those in italic are to captions only (e.g. *123*).